Research and the World Health Organization

A history of the
Advisory Committee on Health Research
1959–1999

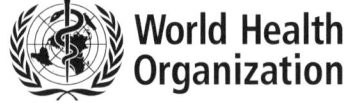

WHO Library Cataloguing-in-Publication Data

Research and the World Health Organization: a history of the Advisory Committee on Health Research, 1959–1999.

1.Research – history. 2.World Health Organization – history. 3.Health services research. 4.Health policy. I.World Health Organization.

ISBN 978 92 4 156411 3   (NLM classification: W 84.3)

© **World Health Organization 2010**

All rights reserved. Publications of the World Health Organization can be obtained from WHO Press, World Health Organization, 20 Avenue Appia, 1211 Geneva 27, Switzerland (tel.: +41 22 791 3264; fax: +41 22 791 4857; e-mail: bookorders@who.int). Requests for permission to reproduce or translate WHO publications – whether for sale or for noncommercial distribution – should be addressed to WHO Press, at the above address (fax: +41 22 791 4806; e-mail: permissions@who.int).

The designations employed and the presentation of the material in this publication do not imply the expression of any opinion whatsoever on the part of the World Health Organization concerning the legal status of any country, territory, city or area or of its authorities, or concerning the delimitation of its frontiers or boundaries. Dotted lines on maps represent approximate border lines for which there may not yet be full agreement.

The mention of specific companies or of certain manufacturers' products does not imply that they are endorsed or recommended by the World Health Organization in preference to others of a similar nature that are not mentioned. Errors and omissions excepted, the names of proprietary products are distinguished by initial capital letters.

All reasonable precautions have been taken by the World Health Organization to verify the information contained in this publication. However, the published material is being distributed without warranty of any kind, either expressed or implied. The responsibility for the interpretation and use of the material lies with the reader. In no event shall the World Health Organization be liable for damages arising from its use.

Designed by minimum graphics
Printed in Malta

Contents

Acknowledgements	vii
Background	vii
Executive Summary	1
1. Introduction	5
2. Statutory background	7
2.1 Definition of WHO research policies by the World Health Assembly and the WHO Executive Board	7
2.2 Functions of the Advisory Committee(s) on Medical Research	9
2.3 Principles of advisory committee (ACMR and ACHR) membership (1959–1998)	10
3. Timeline and milestones	12
3.1 Timeline: the four phases of WHO	12
3.2 Milestones along the way	13
3.2.1 Launching special programmes	17
3.2.2 Promoting health services/systems research	19
3.2.3 Primary health care	21
3.2.4 Critical study of primary health care	23
3.2.5 Milestones in charting research policies and strategies	24
4. Research structures and processes: the means to an end	28
4.1 Documenting disparities in research	28
4.2 Principles of scientific cooperation for WHO	30
4.3 WHO mechanisms for the acquisition of scientific and technical/technological advice	31
4.3.1 Background	31
4.3.2 WHO collaborating centres	31
4.3.3 Functions and role of WHO collaborating centres	32
4.3.4 Pan American Health Organization centres	33
4.4 Research capacity strengthening and the special programmes	34
4.4.1 Infrastructural and managerial problems	34
4.4.2 Prioritizing action research	34
4.4.3 Mechanisms for research capacity strengthening	35

		4.4.4 Developing networks	36
		4.4.5 Research career structures	37
		4.4.6 UNDP/World Bank/WHO Special Programme for Research and Training in Tropical Diseases: research capability strengthening	37
		4.4.7 WHO Special Programme of Research, Development and Research Training in Human Reproduction: strengthening national research capabilities in human reproduction	40
	4.5	Convening major stakeholders in global health	43
5.	**The broad range of WHO's research activities**		**44**
	5.1	Subjects discussed by the ACMR and ACHR	44
	5.2	Forward-looking initiatives in research	44
		5.2.1 Research in epidemiology and communication science	44
		5.2.2 Early warning systems	44
		5.2.3 Geographic information systems	45
		5.2.4 Pattern analysis	46
		5.2.5 Systems analysis	46
		5.2.6 Transfer of technology	49
	5.3	Methodological issues	49
	5.4	Substantive themes	50
	5.5	Initiatives in formulating research strategy, 1950(2000	51
		5.5.1 The Zuckerman roundtable (1975)	52
		5.5.2 Conclusions of the McKeown Report (1988)	53
		5.5.3 The importance of research career structures (technical discussions at the World Health Assembly, 1990)	54
		5.5.4 New methodologies and the need to better understand the economic environment	54
		5.5.5 The impact of scientific advances on future health (1994)	54
		5.5.6 Research policy agenda for science and technology to support global health development (1998)	55
6.	**Regional contributions to health-related research**		**56**
	6.1	WHO AFRICAN REGION	57
		6.1.1 Introduction	57
		6.1.2 Special research programmes	57
		6.1.3 Health research	58
		6.1.4 AACHR support to specific programmes	58
		6.1.5 Sustainability versus brain-drain: a great challenge for Africa	59
		6.1.6 Conclusion	59
	6.2	WHO EASTERN MEDITERRANEAN REGION	60
		6.2.1 The Eastern Mediterranean Advisory Committee for Health Research	60
		6.2.2 Research Policy and Cooperation unit	60

	6.2.3 Promotion of effective health systems in Member States	61
	6.2.4 Research ethics	64
	6.2.5 Web site of the Research Policy and Cooperation unit of the regional office	64
	6.2.6 Conclusion	64
6.3	WHO EUROPEAN REGION	65
	6.3.1 Introduction	65
	6.3.2 Analytical review	65
	6.3.3 A new era	67
	6.3.4 Fit for the future	69
6.4	WHO SOUTH-EAST ASIA REGION	70
	6.4.1 Background	70
	6.4.2 National research capability strengthening	71
	6.4.3 Promotion, coordination and support of regional priority research projects	71
	6.4.4 The role of SEA/ACHR today and in the future	73
6.5	WHO WESTERN PACIFIC REGION	74
	6.5.1 Introduction	74
	6.5.2 History of the Western Pacific Advisory Committee on Medical/Health Research	74
	6.5.3 Health research councils and analogous bodies	75
	6.5.4 The Institute for Medical Research, Kuala Lumpur, as the WHO Regional Centre for Research and Training in Tropical Diseases and Nutrition	76
	6.5.5 WHO collaborating centres	77
	6.5.6 The future	77
6.6	PAN AMERICAN HEALTH ORGANIZATION	78
	6.6.1 Introduction	78
	6.6.2 Strengthening "good" governance and stewardship for research and the national health research systems in Latin American and Caribbean countries	78
	6.6.3 Health research promotion and the common good	80
	6.6.4 Improving competencies for health research	81
	6.6.5 Developing and maintaining sustainable health research systems	81
	6.6.6 Health research alliances and collaboration	83
	6.6.7 Conclusion	84
7. Epilogue		**86**
8. WHO Research for Health Strategy approved by the Sixty-third World Health Assembly 2010		**87**
References		**88**

Annexes 93

Annex 1. Summary of the report of the ACMR Subcommittee on the Enhancement of Transfer of Technology to Developing Countries with Special Reference to Health, 1986   77

Annex 2. The Research policy agenda, 1998 (excerpts)   81

Annex 3. Lord Zuckerman's statement to the 1975 roundtable meeting   88

Annex 4. The final report of Prof. T McKeown, 1988   91

Annex 5. Recommendations from the World Health Assembly technical discussions, 1990   102

Annex 6. Extract from Research for health: principles, perspectives and strategies, 1993   105

Annex 7. Recommendations from the colloquium on "The impact of scientific advances on future health" (excerpts)   108

Annex 8. Summary of the 1998 Research policy agenda for science and technology to support global health development (excerpts)   112

Acknowledgements

WHO gratefully acknowledges the contribution of Dr Pierre Mansourian, who prepared the text of this publication. *Research and the World Health Organization: a history of the Advisory Committee on Health Research 1959–1999* is the product of contributions by a number of persons: WHO Regional Office for Africa: Dr T Nchinda, WHO Regional Office for the Americas/Pan American Health Organization: Dr Ludovic Reveiz and Dr L Gabriel Cuervo, WHO Regional Office for the Eastern Mediterranean: Dr M Afzal, WHO Regional Office for Europe: Professor M Manciaux, WHO Regional Office for South-East Asia: Dr U Ko Ko, Dr Aung Than Batu, WHO Regional Office for the Western Pacific: Dr B Scoggins, Dr A Shirai, Dr M Jegathesan. In addition, Dr Reijo Salmela (then Regional Adviser for Research Policy and Cooperation in the Western Pacific Regional Office) organized the meeting in Manila, Philippines, in November 2007 at which the project to produce this publication was launched.

WHO acknowledges the contribution of the following members of the Advisory Committee on Health Research, who reviewed the draft manuscript: Professor Fred Binka, School of Public Health, University of Ghana, Accra, Ghana; Professor Mahmoud Fathalla, Faculty of Medicine, Assiut University, Assiut, Egypt; and Dr Ana Langer, EngenderHealth, New York,USA.

In addition, the following WHO staff assisted in the preparation of this history: Mr Robert Terry, Mr Christopher Jones and Ms Harin Silalahi, WHO Headquarters, Research Policy and Coordination.

Thanks are also due to Mr David Bramley, who edited the final text.

Above all, WHO expresses its gratitude to the many people who have served on the Advisory Committee on Medical Research/Advisory Committee on Health Research since its establishment in 1959. Their contributions to the work of the Committee, to the policies of WHO and to global developments in health research over the past 50 years have been invaluable.

This publication was supported under a grant from the Bill & Melinda Gates Foundation (grant number 49275.01).

Background

This paper was commissioned to inform the preparation of the development of the WHO Strategy on Research for Health approved by the Sixty-third World Health Assembly in May 2010 within Resolution WHA63.21.

Executive Summary

The Constitution of the World Health Organization (WHO), drawn up in 1946 two years before the Organization formally began operations, includes among WHO's functions "to promote and conduct research in the field of health". While plans for a World Health Research Centre came to nothing, there was considerable pressure from WHO's governing bodies to make the significance of research more overt in WHO's organizational structure.

In 1959, the Advisory Committee on Medical Research (ACMR) was founded and given the role of advising WHO's Director-General on research issues and formulating "global priorities for health research" in the light of policies set by WHO's governing bodies. While the present report traces the contribution of this advisory committee to WHO involvement in research from 1959 to 1999, the committee continues its work to this day. The ACMR was renamed the Advisory Committee on Health Research (ACHR) in 1986.

The Pan American Health Organization (PAHO) set up its own regional advisory committee on medical/health research in the Americas in 1962, and the other five WHO regions followed suit in the 1970s. Described in chapter 6 of this report, the work of these regional ACHRs remains an important feature of WHO's activities and thinking in the field of research.

With the ACMR newly in place, research attracted particular attention from the World Health Assembly, with delegates passing no fewer than 15 World Health Assembly resolutions on health research during the 1960s. These resolutions ensured that research became an important feature of an increasing number of WHO programmes. In 1965, WHO's growing emphasis on research resulted in the establishment in Lyon, France, of the International Agency for Research on Cancer (IARC) as a specialized cancer research centre of WHO.

The 1970s saw the creation of the first "special programme" in WHO – the Special Programme of Research, Development and Research Training in Human Reproduction (HRP) – initiated in 1972. Fifteen years later it became an interagency programme jointly operated by the United Nations Development Programme (UNDP), the United Nations Population Fund (UNFPA), WHO and the World Bank.

The "special programme" model, which looked at an area of health research from a variety of perspectives and united the efforts of several agencies in pursuit of a common research goal, was particularly favoured by ACMR members. In 1974, the ACMR formally recommended the establishment of another special programme – this time on research and training in tropical diseases. Following further ACMR discussions in

1975, the Special Programme for Research and Training in Tropical Diseases (TDR) was founded that year and became operational in 1976. Functioning under the auspices of WHO, TDR was (and is) a joint programme of the United Nations Children's Fund (UNICEF), UNDP and the World Bank.

The ACMR spent a good deal of time and effort in the late 1970s on the aims, objectives and programme components of TDR. The advisory committee recommended, for instance, that the research component of TDR should be global in scope, that there should be external peer review of research projects prior to funding, and that younger scientists should be encouraged – including by furtherance of research career structures). By 1976, ACMR members were urging the establishment of a special programme on health services/systems research, although this idea did not find the kind of support from agencies and donors that HRP and TDR had done.

While strategic thinking played an important role in the ACMR's agenda from the beginning, in the last quarter of the 20th century the ACMR took on a more obviously visionary role. Reflections on future challenges came significantly to the fore in 1975 when Lord Solly Zuckerman chaired a roundtable meeting which examined the processes for defining what kinds of biomedical research programmes should be encouraged at national and international levels. As the next year, WHO's governing bodies discussed WHO's role in health research, with the World Health Assembly passing a resolution (WHA29.64) that stressed the need for a "comprehensive and long-term programme for the development and coordination of biomedical and health services research". That led the ACMR to deliberately focus on "long-term perspectives of WHO's research programme".

As the concept of primary health care developed, the need to expand local capacity for research became self-evident. Regional ACMRs were established and the network of WHO collaborating centres was expanded. Designated by the Director-General of WHO, the collaborating centres support WHO programmes at national and international levels. In addition, a WHO collaborating centre is expected to participate in strengthening country resources – in terms of information, services, research and training – to support national health development. Some regions – notably the Americas and Western Pacific – also identified and strengthened specialist research centres for particular diseases. As the collaborating centres and specialist institutions increased in number, collaboration between them grew and the sharing of knowledge and expertise in research spread in a way that could not have been imagined in earlier decades.

In the late 1970s WHO adopted the Global Strategy for Health for All, based on the principles of primary health care that emerged from the Alma-Ata conference of 1978. By the early 1980s there was growing realization, both within WHO and elsewhere, that a health research strategy was needed to support the health-for-all strategy. In 1983 an ACMR subcommittee was formed specifically to recommend what such a strategy should comprise. The subcommittee, chaired by Professor T McKeown, reported in 1986 and 1988. The report – which was discussed by WHO governing bodies at both global and regional levels – came to the conclusion that achieving health for all meant reaching a level of health below which it was hoped that no country would fall.

One of the issues identified as an obstacle to research was the lack of a career structure for researchers in many countries. When a series of "technical discussions" on research for health for all was held during the Forty-third World Health Assembly in 1990, the need for national research career structures was highlighted by delegates.

By 1993 the ACHR, as it was by then known, called for a better understanding of the economic environment and its effects on health. Referring to the statement in the WHO Constitution that health is "not merely the absence of disease or infirmity", the ACHR emphasized the impact on health of factors such as quality of life, protection against biological and psychosocial damage, the intensity and nature of risks to health, and the presence of health defects and health-relevant deficits. A year later, a colloquium on "The impact of scientific advances on future health" was convened with the aim of identifying the most critical developments in science that were likely to have a major impact on medicine and public health over the following 20 years. Among a variety of topics, the colloquium emphasized DNA technology and this became a major focus of the ACHR as the 1990s progressed – as did changing perspectives of disease and disability (including the concept of disability-adjusted life years, or DALYs), and the impact on public health of the "constructed environment" with its pollution, radiation and electromagnetic fields.

At the end of the 40-year period covered by this report, the ACHR published its *Research policy agenda for science and technology to support global health development* (1998) which tried to identify issues that advisory committee members foresaw as influencing the health research agenda of the third millennium. The advisory committee noted that "whereas the use of advanced technologies is providing people with new opportunities, there is an increase in starvation and misery in many countries". It added that, in spite of diversity, humanity shares a common fate, condition and ethic. As it looked at an increasingly globalizing world in which social indicators were frequently expressed in monetary terms, thus linking happiness to material welfare, the ACHR warned that national data based on averages often do not reveal pockets of poverty or poor health. And in a world where the 4 million scientists and engineers were distributed in a ratio of 25 to 1 between developed and developing countries, members of the ACHR looked forward to an age in which health research could be furthered through a "network of scientific networks" using new communication technologies.

A timeline of the history of the ACMR/ACHR is contained in Table 1. The history of the ACHR in many ways mirrors that of WHO itself. The initial focus on infectious diseases, the shift of emphasis to communities and to primary health care, the strengthening of local capacity, and the challenge of achieving equity in health in a globalized world – these are all major issues that have occupied both the advisory committee and WHO itself. Just who led the way is hard to say. What can be said is that WHO has always needed health research and will continue to need even more in the future.

TABLE 1. **The ACMR/ACHR health research timeline 1959–1999**

YEAR	EVENT
1959	Advisory Committee on Medical Research established by World Health Assembly resolution WHA12.17
1960	World Health Assembly resolution WHA13.64 on the Intensified Programme of Medical Research
1962	Americas Advisory Committee on Medical/Health Research established
1965	Foundation of the International Agency for Research on Cancer (IARC)
1972	Creation of the Special Programme of Research, Development and Research Training in Human Reproduction (HRP)
1975	Creation of the Special Programme for Research and Training in Tropical Diseases (TDR)
1976	African Advisory Committee on Medical/Health Research established
1976	Eastern Mediterranean Advisory Committee on Biomedical Research established (became the Eastern Mediterranean Committee on Health Research in 1982)
1976	European Advisory Committee on Medical/Health Research established
1976	South-East Asia Advisory Committee on Medical/Health Research established
1976	Western Pacific Advisory Committee on Medical/Health Research established
1978	International Conference on Primary Health Care, Alma-Ata, USSR
1979	United Nations Conference on Science and Technology for Development, Vienna
1986	Advisory Committee on Medical Research becomes Advisory Committee on Health Research
1986	Report of the ACHR's Subcommittee on Health Research Strategy published, with an update two years later
1990	Report of the Commission on Health Research for Development estimates that only 5% of global resources for health research are spent on health problems of low and middle-income countries
1990	Technical discussions on research for health during the Forty-third World Health Assembly
1993	Formation of the Council on Health Research for Development (COHRED)
1993	ACHR issues report on *Research for health: principles, perspectives, strategies*
1994	The ACHR and the Council for International Organizations of Medical Sciences (CIOMS) hold joint colloquium on "The impact of scientific advances on future health"
1994	Creation of an ad hoc committee on research for health intervention options
1997	Global Forum on Health Research established
1998	ACHR issues report on *Research policy agenda for science and technology to support global health development*

1. Introduction

The World Health Organization (WHO) is an intergovernmental organization, and is a specialized technical agency of the United Nations. Its constitution came into force on 7 April 1948, a date that is celebrated every year as World Health Day. The founders of the organization, who included Dr. Brock Chisholm (from Canada) who became the first WHO Director-General (1948–1953), saw health as a public good, closely linked to peace and socioeconomic development. They valued a programme of work based on science, research and the acquisition of new knowledge that could be demonstrated as effective. Many present-day concerns about equity, technology utilization and evidence-based policy stem from and build on the earlier WHO vision.

The first 50 years of WHO witnessed many research-related developments that are documented in this report. They include:

- A high-level scientific body called the Advisory Committee on Medical Research (ACMR) was created as early as 1959 to advise WHO's Director-General on matters pertaining to research.
- From the mid-1970s onwards, all WHO regional offices became involved in research and established regional committees on medical research (the Americas Region had its own such committee since 1962).
- Science and technology have been considered the backbone of WHO's activities and were identified as a major programme in WHO's General Programme of Work in the 1970s and 1980s.
- A number of "special programmes" and dedicated research efforts have been promoted in areas such as fertility regulation, tropical diseases and others.
- Several upstream studies have been conducted to find out how best to interlink WHO's research strategies with its main operational activities.
- The advocacy of and focus on primary health care as a means to promote equity and acceptable health levels have characterized WHO's involvement in the health systems domain. During the 1990s, major contributions in the description and understanding of the disease burden amplified WHO's capabilities in this area.
- Ways and means to facilitate technology transfer to developing countries have been articulated through a joint effort of the ACMR and the WHO secretariat. Forward-looking studies in the multisectoral aspects of health were promoted during the 1970s and 1980s.
- New methods, concepts and techniques have been introduced at various times – such as systems analysis (e.g. operations research in tuberculosis control), pattern analysis

(e.g. in the epidemiology of rabies), geographic information systems (e.g. in tropical diseases research) and early warning systems (e.g. in environmental monitoring).
- One of the main tasks has been to cooperate with other United Nations organs in the domain of science and technology, thus helping to assess the disparities in research capacity throughout the world. For example, the "90/10 gap" was well documented for the United Nations Conference on Science and Technology for Development (UNCSTD) in 1979.
- The "convening power" of WHO has been recognized by other major stakeholders in health research, with examples from areas such as AIDS, bovine spongiform encephalopathy (BSE), severe acute respiratory syndrome (SARS), and H5N1 and H1N1 outbreaks.

In the following sections, all these dimensions of WHO's work are described. This overview outlines the statutory background for WHO's research, identifies the milestones in health research over five decades, and discusses issues of both process and programmes. The report also includes accounts of regional efforts in health research.

2. Statutory background

The earliest documents associated with the establishment of WHO show the acceptance of "research" as a function. The original four memoranda submitted by the United Nations members from France, United Kingdom, United States and Yugoslavia, and used by the Technical Preparatory Committee for the International Health Conference (which approved WHO's constitution) of 1946, listed the promotion of research among the proposed functions of the new body. Consequently research as a function was included in chapter II, Article 2 (n) of the constitution which reads "to promote and conduct research in the field of health".

Among the overall functions of the Organization, the constitution also describes the specific functions of the World Health Assembly. With regard to research, the text states that the function of the Health Assembly is "to promote and conduct research in the field of health by the personnel of the Organization, by the establishment of its own institution or by co-operation with official or non-official institution of any Member with the consent of its Government".

The WHO constitution also refers to research among the functions of the WHO Executive Board. Thus, article 28 of the constitution states that the Board is authorized:

> "to take emergency measures within the functions and financial resources of the Organization to deal with events requiring immediate action. In particular it may authorize the Director-General to take the necessary steps to combat epidemics, to participate in the organization of health relief to victims of a calamity and to undertake studies and research the urgency of which has been drawn to the attention of the Board by any member or by the Director-General."

Thus the constitutional authority for WHO in the field of research is far-reaching and must be understood in the context of the philosophical framework of the constitution which is based on the cooperation of WHO's Member States for promoting and protecting world health. This is notwithstanding a debate around the very concept of health (see Box 1).

2.1 Definition of WHO research policies by the World Health Assembly and the WHO Executive Board

As early as 1949, the second World Health Assembly approved the basic principles that would guide WHO's research. These were expressed in Resolution WHA2.19, as follows:

> **BOX 1**
>
> ### Defining health: three different perspectives
>
> "Health is a state of complete physical, mental and social well-being and not merely the absence of disease or infirmity"
> *(Preamble to WHO's Constitution, 1948).*
>
> "Health, like happiness, cannot be defined in exact measurable terms because its presence is so largely a matter of subjective judgement. About as precise as one can get is that health is a relative affair that represents the degree to which an individual can operate with effectiveness within the particular circumstances of his heredity and his physical and cultural environment. Definitions that embrace the concept of 'the absence of disease' in reality are misleading. For all living things are diseased."
> *(Professor W McDermott, former member of the ACMR. Human ecology and human disease. In: Human Ecology and Public Health, Macmillan, 1969).*
>
> This logo was developed and adopted by the ACHR in preparing papers for the World Health Assembly Technical Discussions on Health Research in 1990. The symbol represents the population explosion witnessed during the 20th century (middle curve) which divides (on the left) high infant and continuing mortality from the goal of ACHR which was increased survival for all age groups (on the right).
>
>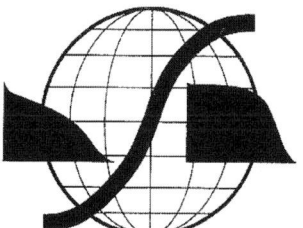

"… whereas the development of planned programmes requires continuous application of research and investigation of many problems, the solution of which may be found essential for the diagnosis, treatment and prevention of disease, and for the promotion of positive health;

Whereas research includes field investigations as well as those conducted in laboratories,

The Second World Health Assembly resolves that the following guiding principles should be applied in the organization of research under the auspices of the World Health Organization:

(1) research and coordination of research are essential functions of the World Health Organization;
(2) first priority should be given to research directly related to the programmes of the World Health Organization;
(3) research should be supported in existing institutions and should form part of the duties of field teams supported by the World Health Organization;
(4) all locally supported research should be so directed as to encourage assumption of responsibility for its continuance by local agencies where indicated;
(5) the World Health Organization should not consider at the present time the establishment, under its own auspices, of international research institutions."

This resolution represents the basic Health Assembly policy on research. Although subsequent resolutions,[1] have emphasized certain new and perhaps revolutionary aspects concerning the modalities of cooperation and coordination, they have not changed the policy foundations for WHO's involvement in research.

Certain implications of the resolution should be noted. Besides accepting the contribution that research may make to WHO's progress, the resolution gives two important policy directives. First, it requires that research undertaken by WHO should be related directly to the Organization's work. This is indicative of the converse wish that research outside the areas of concern of WHO programmes should not be given high priority, if supported at all. Secondly, the last three points give a clear direction of methods and approaches to be followed. Encouragement, support and coordination of research in local institutions and teams – rather than the creation, building and support of special internationally administered and staffed establishments – were thereby set early on as WHO principles.

2.2 Functions of the Advisory Committee(s) on Medical Research

In 1958, an "intensified research programme" was proposed, followed in 1959 by the setting up, under World Health Assembly resolution WHA12.17, of the Advisory Committee on Medical Research (ACMR) and the Special Account for Medical Research (1).

The main functions of the ACMR were described as:

— to advise the Director-General of WHO on the general orientation of WHO's research;
— to advise on the formulation of global priorities for health research in the light of the policies set by the World Health Assembly and the WHO Executive Board and on the basis of regional priorities evolved in response to the health problems of the countries;
— to review research activities, monitor their execution and evaluate their results, from the standpoint of scientific and technical policy;
— to formulate ethical criteria applicable to these research activities;
— to take a prominent part in the harmonization of WHO's research efforts between the country, regional and interregional levels, and in their effective global synthesis.

Regional Advisory Committees on Medical Research were established during the 1970s and, although the specific terms of reference differ according to the needs and conditions of the regions, their broad functions can be summarized as follows:

- They advise the regional director on the formulation of policies for the development of health research in the region, in accordance with directives provided by the gov-

---

[1] Notably resolutions WHA11.35, WH12.17, WHA18.43, WHA19.34, WHA25.60, WHA26.42, WHA27.61, WHA28.70, WHA 29.64, WHA30.40, WHA31.35 and WHA32.15.

erning bodies (World Health Assembly, Executive Board and regional committees) and within the framework of the global WHO policy. This formulation includes the identification of national and regional priorities.
- They establish mechanisms for coordinating research at national, intraregional and interregional levels.
- They develop research potential and capability, nationally and regionally.
- They evaluate the regional research programme in terms of stated objectives and the mechanisms employed.
- They harmonize regional research activities with the activities of other regions and with WHO headquarters, in close collaboration with the global ACMR.

Whereas the governing bodies have a constitutional responsibility to establish policy guidelines for WHO's programme (including research), the role of the ACMRs is mainly to assist the WHO secretariat in translating such guidelines into action. This implies a broad spectrum of efforts ranging from the analysis and articulation of research policies to the definition of specific research themes having appropriate disciplinary and geographical configurations.

In 1976, the global ACMR suggested 10 criteria for selecting priority areas for WHO research (Box 2).[1]

2.3 Principles of advisory committee (ACMR and ACHR) membership (1959–1998)

Members were appointed in a personal capacity by the Director-General for a period of up to four years (not immediately renewable). The Director-General accepted recommendations from the chair, the regional directors, the Deputy Director-General, the Assistant Director-General, WHO departmental directors, and the secretary of the advisory committee.

The membership sought to achieve an equitable representation of gender, disciplines and regions. The advisory committee has counted prestigious names in its membership: Nobel laureates and influential figures in biomedical, public health and/or clinical sciences.[2]

No fewer than 18 Nobel laureates have been members of the ACMR/ACHR, one of whom was also the founder of WHO's immunology unit (N.K. Jerne).

---

[1] The Advisory Committee on Medical Research (ACMR) was renamed Advisory Committee on Health Research (ACHR) in 1986, by decision of the World Health Assembly.

[2] Chairs of the ACMR and ACHR during the period under review were: A.J. Wallgreen (1959–1963), R. Courrier (1964–1967), Lord Rosenheim (1968–1972), N. Scrimshaw (1973–1977), S. Bergstrom (1978–1982), V. Ramalingaswami (1983–1986), B.O. Osuntokun (1987–1989), M. Gabr (1990–1993), T. Fliedner (1994–1998).

BOX 2

Proposed criteria for selecting priority areas for WHO research (ACMR, 1976)

Selection of priority areas for health research should be based on the following criteria:

i. The magnitude of the problem, especially in the developing countries.

ii. The suitability of the problem for international collaborative research efforts coordinated by WHO.

iii. The priority of the problem as perceived by individual countries themselves.

iv. The relevance of the problem to the socioeconomic development of Member States.

v. The probability of finding solution (or important clarifications) and the feasibility of applying them nationally, including the time and costs required.

vi. The availability of manpower, facilities and funds to carry out the research to ensure as far as possible the achievement of significant results.

vii. The involvement of the countries themselves, especially their scientific communities and facilities, in the research efforts to be undertaken preferably where the problem exists, so as to upgrade national research capabilities.

viii. The level of ongoing research efforts, both nationally and internationally, to solve the problem.

ix. The benefit which would accrue from the application of the results of successful research efforts, especially in the developing countries.

x. The potential usefulness of the results of the research in the solution of other problems.

3. Timeline and milestones

3.1 Timeline: the four phases of WHO

In this review the first 50 years of WHO have been subdivided into four phases: a "growth phase", an "advocacy phase", an "accountancy phase" and a "recalibration phase" (*2*).

The first growth phase corresponds to the period of leadership of Dr. Marcolino Candau who assumed four successive mandates as Director-General between 1953 and 1973.

In the early 1950s, WHO had a budget of 5 million and some 100 staff at its headquarters in Geneva. Twenty years later, the staff had multiplied 10-fold and the budget approximately 20 times. Dr. Candau was profoundly convinced of the role of science and research in the life of WHO, and attempted to create a World Health Research Centre. Several documents relate to the planning of such a centre (*3*).

The initial design mutated into several entities, namely the WHO Division of Research in Epidemiology and Communication Science (RECS), the International Agency for Research on Cancer (IARC) and the International Drug-Monitoring Network. A series of World Health Assembly resolutions throughout the 1960s reflects the intense degree of involvement with research-related issues (cf 3.2 below).

The advocacy phase began with Dr. Halfdan Mahler (Director-General between 1973 and 1988), who had been deeply influenced by a 10-year period of fieldwork in India. He promoted the "operationalization" of research, implying:

— immediate emphasis on health services and health systems research;
— the regionalization of research, which started in the mid-1970s;
— prompting the ACMR to elaborate research strategies congruent with the global "Health for All" strategy;
— the encouragement of large-scale "special programmes" for research and training, inspired by research and development in human reproduction. The pattern of tropical disease research was followed in the areas of diarrhoeal diseases, acute respiratory infections, AIDS, vaccine technology, health systems research, mental health, toxicology etc.

Despite the intention to operationalize, the role of WHO in most of these endeavours was more one of promotion and advocacy.

The accountancy phase refers principally to "best buys". WHO was becoming increasingly dependent on extrabudgetary funds. Donor agencies were anxious to see a unified strategy with clear measurable targets and cost-effective interventions, while WHO was seen as dispersing its resources and duplicating efforts. All this had implications for research. A first initiative came from the Independent Commission on Health Research for Development which carried out a study between 1987 and 1989 and issued its report in 1990 (*4*). This was the year of "Technical Discussions" on research at the World Health Assembly (*5*). Two important prescriptions emerged: the notion of "essential national health research" (ENHR), and the need to allocate 2% of national health expenditure for ENHR. The next intervention was the creation of the Council on Health Research for Development (COHRED), an NGO whose role was to bring together all stakeholders to promote ENHR (*6*). Then in 1993 the World Bank's *World development report*, which was devoted to "investing in health" (*7*), for the first time made use of the metric of disability-adjusted life years (DALYs) to document the global burden of disease (*8*).[1] This gave rise in 1994 to the creation of an Ad Hoc Committee on Health Research related to future intervention options, which reviewed the financing needs across the spectrum of health research and determined the best buys (*9*). Finally, as part of the institutional arrangements derived from the ad hoc study, the Global Forum for Health Research was created as a Swiss-based foundation in 1997 (*10*).

The fourth phase is called the recalibration phase because WHO has moved to resize, reshape and reorient since 1998 as a preeminent player (though not necessarily the predominant one) in the arena of global health. Although this phase extends beyond the period covered by this historical review, it would start with major and far-reaching initiatives, such as the *World health report 2000* and the report of the Commission on Macroeconomics and Health (the Sachs report), both of which attracted great attention and scrutiny worldwide.

3.2 Milestones along the way

The 1960s can be remembered by a stream of landmark World Health Assembly resolutions related to research, notably on:

— the Intensified Programme of Medical Research (Resolution WHA13.64, 1960);
— the International Encouragement of Scientific Research into the Control of Cancerous Diseases (Resolution WHA14.54, 1961);
— the Smallpox Eradication Programme (Resolution WHA 15.53, 1962);
— the Clinical and Pharmacological Evaluation of Drugs (Resolution WHA15.41, 1962);
— the Development of the Malaria Eradication Programme (Resolution WHA17.22, 1964);
— the Establishment of an International Registry for Research on Cancer (Resolution WHA18.44, 1965);
— the Adverse Drug Reaction Monitoring System (Resolution WHA18.42, 1965);

---

[1] At the turn of the century, about 20% of global DALYs lost were due to lower respiratory infections, perinatal conditions, diarrhoeal diseases and HIV/AIDS. Projections for 2020 describe a different picture, with major causes of the disease burden being ischaemic heart disease (5.9%) unipolar major depression (5.7%), motor vehicle accidents (5.1%) and cerebrovascular disease (4.4%). In terms of risk factors, malnutrition has been shown to account for about 16% of the global disease burden, while poor water supply and sanitation account for about 7%.

- the Programme Activities in the Health Aspects of World Population which might be developed by WHO (Resolution WHA18.49, 1965);
- the Compendium of Recommendations, Definitions and Standards relating to Health Statistics (Resolution WHA20.19, 1967);
- Health and Economic Development (Resolution WHA20.53, 1967);
- Health Aspects of Population Dynamics (Resolution WHA21.43, 1968);
- Re-examination of the Global Strategy of Malaria Eradication (WHA22.39, 1969);
- Research on Methods of Vector Control (Resolution WHA22.40, 1969);
- the Question of General and Complete Disarmament: Chemical and Bacteriological (Biological) weapons and the Consequences of their Possible Use (Resolution WHA22.58, 1969);
- the United Nations Conference on the Human Environment (Resolution WHA22.57, 1969).

The 1970s were marked by the historical decision of Director-General Mahler to decentralize research in order to strengthen national capacities in health-related research. Some institutions sought to become centres of excellence and succeeded (see Box 3).

BOX 3

Features that determine the success of a research institution

The ideal research institution

Based on studies carried out by the ACHR, the main features which determine the success and sustainability of a research institution include: (i) a history of consistently strong leadership, dedication to quality work and constant improvement; (ii) a tradition of scientific inquiry coupled with a sense of discipline and rigour in research management; (iii) systematic documentation of professional and research activities, including publications; (iv) a critical mass, in professional, technical and financial terms, to guarantee momentum; (v) and environment conducive to research and likely to motivate young scientist; (vi) a close relationship with policy planners and decision makers; and (vii) external cooperation and networking to attract further technical support and funding from international sources.

Furthermore, regional ACMRs and ACHRs have contributed to the definition of regional research priorities (see Table 2), mainly through joint meetings with national medical research councils and analogous bodies (*11*). In several regions, specific projects were undertaken in the areas of strengthening research capacity, including research management, training and methodology, and research career structures (see Table 2). The Director-General and the ACMR also encouraged the formation of special programmes (see Box 4 and Section 3.2.1).

The 1980s saw the ACMR (renamed ACHR in 1986) involved in the formulation of a research strategy (also called the McKeown report) to relate research to the WHO strategy for health for all (*12*). Another major effort was carried out by an ACHR committee working on the transfer of health technology to developing countries

TABLE 2. **Priorities of regional advisory committees on medical/health research (1976–1999)**

		AFRICA	AMERICAS	EASTERN MEDITERRANEAN	EUROPE	SOUTH-EAST ASIA	WESTERN PACIFIC
A	Health services research	X	X	X	X	X	X
	Health care delivery		X	X	X	X	
	Economic aspects of health care		X		X		
	Adequate use of health services		X		X		
	Studies on different health services systems		X		X		
	Health planning and evaluation		X		X		
	Interrelationship between scientific research and health care delivery	X		X			
	Educational research aspects of health manpower development	X	X	X	X	X	
B	Communicable diseases	X	X	X		X	X
	Schistosomiasis	X	X	X		X	X
	Leprosy	X	X	X		X	X
	Malaria	X	X	X		X	X
	Filariasis	X	X			X	X
	Dengue haemorrhagic fever		X			X	X
	Enteric diseases		X				X
	Trypanosomiasis	X	X	X			
	Leishmaniasis	X	X	X			
	Onchocerciasis	X	X	X			
	Diarrhoeal diseases, including cholera		X	X		X	
	Soil-transmitted helminths (ascariasis, hookworm)	X		X			
	Mycotic infection		X	X			
	Tuberculosis		X	X		X	X
	Eye disease (trachoma, conjunctivitis)			X			
C	Chronic liver diseases, including liver cancer		X			X	
D	Population genetics in relation to disease					X	
E	Cardiovascular disease		X				X
	Rheumatic fever		X				X
	Rheumatic heart disease		X				X
	Atherosclerosis						X
	Hypertension		X				X

TABLE 2. Continued

		AFRICA	AMERICAS	EASTERN MEDITERRANEAN	EUROPE	SOUTH-EAST ASIA	WESTERN PACIFIC
F	Family health	X	X	X		X	X
	Maternal and child health	X	X				X
	Family planning		X				X
	Nutrition	X	X	X		X	X
G	Prevention, prophylaxis and early detection		X		X		
H	Evaluation of drugs and other therapeutic and diagnostic substances			X	X	X	
I	Traditional medicine	X				X	
J	Environmental health	X	X			X	X
K	Standards of methods, measurements and terminology in biomedical and health services research		X		X		

BOX 4

The ACMR recommendation on research and training in tropical diseases (June 1974)

Conceiving the Special Programme for Research and Training in Tropical Diseases

After discussing working paper ACMR 16/74.5, the ACMR recommended the institution of an expanded WHO programme for research and training related to tropical communicable diseases and agreed that the objectives of the expanded programme should be:

a) the application of modern biomedical concepts and methods to develop new approaches for the prevention, diagnosis and treatment of communicable tropical diseases;

b) the creation of expertise in the relevant biomedical sciences in developing countries: the emphasis should be placed first on Africa but, building on the experience gained, this aspect of the programme should be extended to other regions as rapidly as available resources allowed;

c) the provision of research training in developing countries in close cooperation with universities and allied institutions and the improvement of career opportunities for research workers;

d) the instigation of continuing studies of the demographic and socioeconomic impact of these diseases and disease control measures developed against them.

> **BOX 5**
>
> **Summary of WHO-related research events, 1988–98**
>
> Developments in health research 1988–98
>
> 1988 – ACHR strategy, final conclusions of the McKeown report
> 1990 – Report of the Commission on Health Research for Health Development
> 1990 – World Health Assembly technical discussions on Research for Health for All
> 1993 – World Bank report on health-wide use of the DALY metric
> 1993 – Formation of the Council on Health Research for Development (COHRED)
> 1993 – ACHR report on *Research for health: principles, perspectives, strategies*
> 1994 – Establishment of ad hoc Committee on research for health intervention options
> 1997 – Establishment of Global Forum on Health Research
> 1998 – ACHR report on *Research policy agenda for science and technology to support global health development*

(*13,14,15,16* and *17*). These issues are described in more detail in section 5.

The 1990s witnessed parallel developments within WHO as well as elsewhere. Following the World Health Assembly's technical discussions on "Research for Health for All" in 1990 (*5*), the ACHR pursued its work on strategies, issuing its 1993 report on *Research for health: principles, perspectives, strategies* (*18*). This was further refined and developed during the decade – namely as the *Research policy agenda for science and technology to support global health development* (*19*).

Some major events (1988–98) relevant to WHO-related research are listed in Box 5.

3.2.1 Launching special programmes

The mid-1970s witnessed the expansion of the "special programme" concept inspired by the programme known as HRP which dealt with research and development in human reproduction biology and epidemiology. HRP had started as an "intensified" programme in fertility regulation, reflecting WHO's dual involvement with biomedical sciences and population health. In 1972, it became the "Special Programme of Research, Development and Research Training in Human Reproduction", attracting substantial extrabudgetary funding.

The Special Programme for Research and Training in Tropical Diseases (TDR) was next, and the rationale of TDR – national capacity-strengthening, focus on applied and multidisciplinary research, interagency cooperation – was followed in the areas of diarrhoeal diseases, acute respiratory infections, AIDS, vaccine technology, health systems research, mental health, toxicology, and others.

A classic example of ACMR's involvement in the creation of a special programme was the case of TDR. At its June 1974 session, the ACMR formally recommended the creation of such a programme (Box 4). The following year (1975), substantive discussions took place again on the programme, and in June 1976 the first operational TDR Director (Dr. A. Lucas) reported back to the ACMR.

The Committee noted that 1976 was a year of planning and pilot activities, and that a meeting of participants would be held in December 1976 to finalize the administrative structure of TDR, and to extend the base of financial support. If the outcome of that meeting was successful, the phase of definitive operation could begin on 1 April 1977.

The ACMR strongly endorsed the two main aims of TDR, namely:

— to provide new weapons to fight tropical diseases and to optimize use of existing weapons;
— to promote self-reliance in problem-solving within developing countries by strengthening research training and institutions.

Both were essential components, mutually dependent and reinforcing. The training should not be regarded simply as a spin-off from the research, the ACMR members said. For this reason, both WHO and the involved Member States should pay special attention to appropriate career structures for the trainees.

In order to achieve its objectives (namely the conquest of the six diseases) a balanced programme was required with short-, medium- and long-term components, and these were discussed in great detail by the ACMR.

The ACMR reaffirmed the need for outside peer review of research projects prior to funding (implicit in the scientific working group mechanism). It also urged that mechanisms be developed for inviting research proposals, particularly from younger scientists, who might provide original ideas in the field. It noted that its members, as individuals, might serve as promoters of the programme in their own countries and regions, both with respect to the involvement of scientists, and with governments and agencies responsible for funding policies.

The ACMR endorsed the concept of a global programme since diseases do not respect national boundaries or WHO regions. The research component should be global in scope from the outset, the ACMR said, and the membership of the scientific working groups should be drawn from all over the world. The training and institution-strengthening component should have Africa as its initial focus, but should become progressively more global as the programme developed. The work would constantly take into account the intimate relationships between parasitic disease, nutritional problems and defence mechanisms in the human host.

The ACMR considered the special programme to be one of the most important activities of WHO and a model for the future, with additional major disease groups incorporated into the special programme once it was thoroughly established. The Committee strongly affirmed the need for minimum funding of US$ 20 million per year for a minimum of 10 years, and urged responsible authorities to respond as generously as possible.

The organizational capacity for change and adaptation to new scientific developments during the 1970s and 1980s was exemplified by the creation of a dedicated WHO unit (Safety Measures in Microbiology, under Dr. V. R. Oviatt), to follow up on the Asilomar Conference on Recombinant DNA (1975), and the creation of the Global Programme on AIDS (January 1987, under Dr. J. Mann). This effort attracted 50 million in the first six months of its life. WHO's attraction of (and dependence on) extrabudgetary funds increased substantially during this period (see Figure 1).

FIG. 1 **The growth of WHO's reliance on extrabudgetary funds over a 10-year period (shown for illustration)**

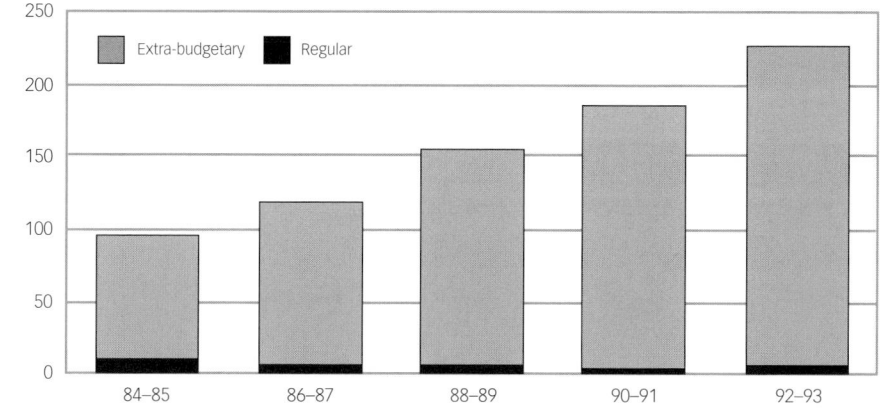

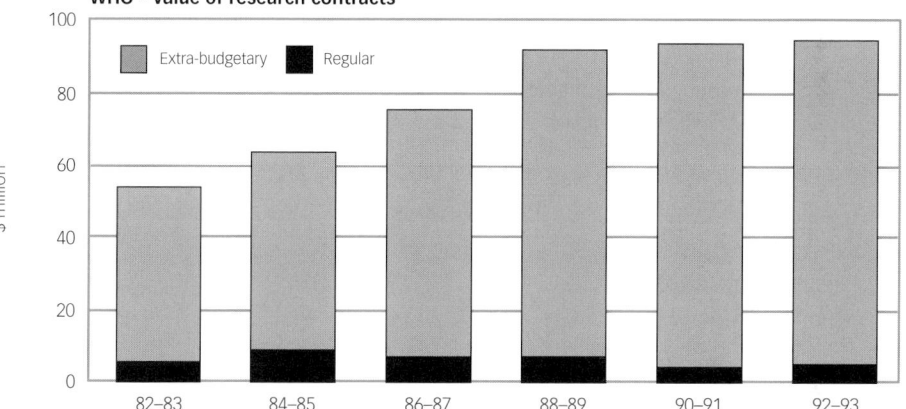

3.2.2 *Promoting health services/systems research*

The 18th session of the ACMR (June 1976) urged that a specific programme in health services/systems research (known as HSR) be developed as soon as possible. This was prompted not only by the Director-General's introductory remarks in 1974, but also by several interventions at meetings of WHO's governing bodies in the early 1970s.

An informal consultation was held in June 1976 before the ACMR with the following terms of reference:

— to formulate a working definition of HSR and define its scope;
— to suggest a WHO policy for research in health services development;
— to define the priority areas on which research in health services development should concentrate;
— to propose new or improved mechanisms by which appropriate action could be defined, promoted, coordinated, planned, implemented and evaluated, both in Member States and WHO;

BOX 6

ACMR recommendations (June 1976) for a special programme on health services/systems research

The ACMR made the following recommendations on health services/systems research in 1976

(a) Immediate formation by the Director-General within WHO of a planning group with adequate representation from the regions and a full-time secretariat to formulate a special programme in HSR. This group should have:
  i. clearly identified tasks;
  ii. a reliable time-frame;
  iii. adequate resources.

(b) The task of this group might include activities such as:
  i. collection of information on the activities of the regional ACMRs and related task forces in the area of HSR;
  ii. assessment of current WHO activities in HSR and of national activities in HSR in which WHO collaborates;
  iii. collation of information on national activities and national capabilities in HSR obtained from countries by the regional offices;
  iv. indication of priorities for future WHO activities in HRS based on analysing country needs as expressed by the countries and by the regional ACHRs and task forces; this could be based, among other factors, on the frequency with which a problem is identified by the countries;
  v. formulation of a special programme for WHO activities in HSR, including the development of a plan of nation with identification of training needs (the methodology available for medium-term programming should be followed);
  vi. preparation of background material for a meeting of donor agencies to be convened by the Director-General to seek funds for implementing the special programme and supporting HSR in countries;
  vii. implementation of the special programme. It is clear that the implementation of the programme will be decentralized with well-identified global functions performed centrally (regional offices, headquarters). These may include mobilization of extra-budgetary resources, methodological improvements, interregional communication and coordination, dissemination of information, etc.;
  viii. keeping the regional ACMRs and their task forces on HSR fully informed of the progress of the planning.

(c) A suggested time frame for these tasks should include:
  i. preparation of an initial report within four months from regions which have not already provided such a report, identifying a number of research projects suitable for early implementation;
  ii. draft of a plan for the special programme within six months and circulation of the plan to potential donors;
  iii. donors meeting within 12 months (before the next section of the ACHR);
  iv. initiation of the special programme on HSR within 18 months.

(d) financial resources for this WHO planning group should be adequate to implement the following:
  i. recruit temporary advisors on a full-time basis for the required period of time;
  ii. arrange meetings with regional and country representatives;
  iii. perform site visits;
  iv. undertake information processing and analysis;
  v. prepare the report.

— to consolidate the results of the discussions into a set of recommendations to the Director-General and the 18th ACMR on the course of action to be taken in the area of HSR in the context of the overall WHO programme.

The meeting was chaired by Dr. K.N. Rao, Director of the Indian Academy of Medical Sciences, with D.O. Anderson of the University of British Columbia as rapporteur, and was attended by several ACMR members, including Sir Douglas Black (who submitted a paper entitled "Priorities in biomedical research: indices of burden", reprinted from *British Medical Journal of Preventive and Social Medicine* (20).

A report discussing the basic principles of HSR was then prepared and presented to the 18th session of the ACMR in June 1976 which endorsed it. The report included a definition of HSR as "the systematic investigation and evaluation of specific aspects relative to the development and functioning of health services in terms of their relationships with health related factors". The definition also expanded on the contextual and disciplinary implications of the term.

The following year (June 1977), another consultation was held under the chairmanship of Mrs Nita Barrow of the Christian Medical Commission, with Prof. K.W. Newell from Wellington, New Zealand, as rapporteur. The ACMR made recommendations concerning the development of a special programme in HSR with the immediate establishment of a planning and implementation group. The full text of the ACMR recommendations is reproduced in Box 6.

Nearly 10 years later (1986), a heated ACMR intervention by Dr Mahler reflected on the Director-General's own assessment of the trials and tribulations of HSR in WHO-related activities. Dr Mahler admitted that WHO seemed to be making no progress in HSR and suggested that the Organization's Member States were more interested in all kinds of "fanciful stupidities" rather than in understanding their own predicaments. A transcript of Dr Mahler's intervention is reproduced in Box 7.

3.2.3 Primary health care

Primary health care has remained for the last 30 years the main global priority for research and development in health care systems, especially in less developed countries. The main tenets can be summarized as follows:

- **Promotion of a healthy lifespan.** Adding years to life may not be an end in itself, but life expectancy (e.g. 70 years) may be a positive surrogate indicator, while survival disparities is a negative one.
- **Universal access to an agreed upon set of essential health care services** including health education, promotion, access to clinical treatment, essential surgery, essential drugs, dental and mental health services (defined in some detail).
- **Survival and health development of children and young people.** Targets may include low infant mortality rates (IMR) (e.g. IMR < 25 per 1000 live births), appropriate weight for height and age, and high immunization rates (e.g. >98%).
- **Health and well-being of women.** Actions range from insurance of maternal health and safety to empowerment of women in the home, education, health system, workplace, and in policy and decision making.

BOX 7

The Director-General's comments on health systems research at the ACHR in 1986

Transcript of Dr Mahler's intervention on health systems research in 1987

"You were trying to provoke me a moment ago, as soon as Professor Robbins came to yet another disastrous failure of health systems research. I feel that I have been whipping that horse now consistently for about 25 years in this organization after coming here to headquarters from India. I don't know what more can be done but we just are not making any real significant progress in this field. And it is very hard to understand that when everybody knows if you have to put a man on the moon you have to make use of that kind of systems research, operations research, whatever you want to call it. And particularly to bring him back again, if anything should happen. And it is very hard for me to understand that nobody in the scientific community cares, after having done a clinical trial on beta-blockers and you find that so-and-so much different should happen if they took the beta-blockers with such-and-such regularity and such-and-such doses. Then nobody cares whether you have a compliance rate of ten or of ninety. And I can go to any amount of countries, in Uruguay I know, and some of them very big and very powerful, where the only thing they said in the Ministry of Health recently when they found that it was about 25%, " well, you know that's people's behaviour ". But I think it is an absolutely incredible waste of resources. And I think it is very unfair to the patients themselves or to whatever health individuals you call people having hypertension. That you don't care about whether they take their drugs or they don't take their drugs. And we all know that this can be radically changed, as in a place like Norway for instance, where they have a very solid kind of operations research group, and they have got it up from about 30% up to about 90%, by doing a few kind of solid kind of studies on how to get the support structure in order …

… So I am simply perhaps masochistically saying really I am very sad that we are so slow. When Professor Brotherstone came here about 25 years ago, he got the most cynical reception that anybody has got from the ACMR, who just simply laughed him out of this room, or another room wherever it was, that this has nothing to do with research and he should not waste such nonsense on prestigious members of ACMR. At least now there has been a change, everybody speaks about health systems research and the regional commissions, advisory committees speak about it and its blah-blahing all over the place. I think it is very sad that Member States are making use of WHO's resources to do all kind of fanciful stupidities like buying a little bit of DDT or cars, or sending a fellow here and there, rather than making use of them in order to get down to understand their own predicament. Because that is the only thing you develop. That is getting out of the old envelope and getting into your own new envelope, not imposed envelopes from the outside. But some envelopes you have developed for yourself. And health systems research is an admirable tool for that".

- **Healthy population development.** This may include healthy and responsible relationships and access to family planning information and services that are culturally acceptable and legal.
- **Elimination of specific endemic diseases or local conditions of ill health.** Targets may be set to control malaria, tuberculosis, tetanus and HIV/AIDS that especially threaten the population (e.g. tetanus incidence = 0).
- **Reduction of avoidable disabilities.** These may include promotion of safety and healthy activity, as well as provision of rehabilitative services to victims of accidents (e.g. road traffic) and disease (e.g. leprosy) as well as coverage of elderly citizens in a naturally aging population.
- **Improvement of nutritional status.** Targets may aim at food supply, avoidance of under-or-over-nutrition, and elimination of micronutrient deficiencies (e.g. vitamin A).
- **Universal access to safe water and healthy environmental living conditions.** Targets might include protected drinking water access (e.g. initially 95%), excreta disposal, and community-defined basic housing, as well as measurable reductions in violence in the community.
- **Healthy lifestyle and behaviour.** Quantifiable actions and outcomes include numbers and types of health promotion activities, targeted access to education, and availability of information and social activity to enhance healthy living and to decrease health damaging behaviour.

3.2.4 Critical study of primary health care

Primary health care and the Global Strategy for Health for All have been the subject of a number of analytical reviews. One of the most perceptive, entitled "An economic evaluation of Health for All" was published by M. Patel in 1986 (*21*). It questioned whether the goals of the strategy were merely a list of ad hoc ideals or whether they were indeed potential building blocks of an implementable global plan. It further specified that traditional planning processes could be represented as (i) defining "policies" in order to (ii) quantify the "resources" needed to (iii) finance the "activities" necessary to (iv) achieve the desired "outcomes".

Patel considered that the 12 target indicators of the strategy could be neatly classified into four logical components of the planning process, namely:

- The first two goals (national endorsement of the policy, and mobilization of community and interest groups) are concerned with policy formation.
- The next four goals (>5% of gross national product [GNP] to health, emphasis on basic care, equitable distribution of staff and resources, international aid support) deal with the resources needed to finance the strategy and the distribution of these resources.
- The activity goals (safe water for all, immunization coverage, local health care for all, maternal and child health) constitute the next stage of a rational planning process for resource allocation.
- The outcome goals (nutrition coverage, IMR <50/1000, life expectancy >60 years,

literacy >70%, GNP per capita >US$ 500) were not seen, however, to match with the consistent nature of the strategy in terms of the relationships between policies, resources and activities.

The critique argued that the desired outcomes were often unlikely to result from the activities proposed. For example, although labour productivity has been linked to health status, it would be futile to argue that major increases in GNP could be achieved by health policy alone. Adult literacy rates were unresponsive to measures proposed by the strategy, but there was some evidence for the reverse. There have also been indications of a relationship between IMR and female literacy as well as GNP per head. However, specific activities to increase literacy or GNP are not part of the core of the strategy.

The paper presented data on the numbers of countries that had at that time achieved the outcome goals (in 1983, none of the low-income countries). It also evaluated the numbers of countries that "might" achieve the outcome goals by 2000, as well as those that were "unlikely" to do so (31 low-income countries).

The analysis enquired to what extent the WHO measure of progress, based on numbers of countries, compared with a measure based on percentages of the world's population. The evidence presented showed some disparities in most categories (already achieved, could be achieved, unlikely to be achieved). It was shown that, although 39% of the world's countries had achieved the IMR goal, this amounted to only 30% of the world's population. Conversely, although 53% of countries had achieved the life expectancy goal, over 63% of the world population had done so.

The argument was further illustrated by the fact that, on a straight count of countries, improvements in the health of an inhabitant of Bhutan (population of about 1 million) would effectively count for 1000 times more progress than improvement in the health of an inhabitant of China (>1 billion).

It may be appropriate to conclude these observations on primary health care by noting that the *World health report 1998* mentioned that the two main goals of WHO's strategy (IMR and life expectancy) had been achieved in all but seven countries. The rate of progress in achieving these goals, as reported by WHO and UNICEF, is still a matter of debate in the public health literature.

3.2.5 *Milestones in charting research policies and strategies*

A first effort in formal strategic thinking and "horizon scanning" was made in June 1975 (17th session) by an ACMR roundtable chaired by Lord S. Zuckerman (*11*).

Important observations emerged. A first generalization was that WHO concerned itself with the encouragement of "worthwhile research". The meeting had been reminded by the Director-General Mahler how much the scientific community suffered from the impression that a vast amount of what was designated research was of poor quality, and that some hardly justified the description. A second generalization was that there were certain problems in the field which could be tackled only internationally (i.e. under the auspices of WHO). Other considerations included the question of constraints, such as barriers to the acceptance of new ideas, and limited resources. The problem of priorities was perceived in dynamic terms (e.g. whether it was possible for the ranking order of initiatives in research to parallel the ranking order of health needs). A premonitory statement was made: "Time is not on our side. Population is growing. Poverty is growing. Urbanization is bringing about new environmental problems. In some countries there appears to be a beginning of breakdown of institutional order. In these circumstances it becomes more and more difficult to transfer knowledge which, if applied, would help to achieve the objectives of WHO."

The ACMR recognized that WHO's research activities had been planned and carried out, with few exceptions, as integral parts of the organization's programmes and not as part of an "organization-wide programme of research coordinated and funded through an identifiable framework and plan".

In 1976, it was estimated that about US$ 5 million representing less than 4% of WHO's regular budget were allocated each year to research activities. Additional extrabudgetary funds estimated at US$ 15 million comprised the remainder of WHO's annual expenditure for research. These modest resources, through their association with WHO programmes, were seen to have a catalytic effect which substantially increased their impact.

The late 1970s saw WHO involved mostly with primary health care and the related Alma Ata Conference, as well as the United Nations Conference on Science and Technology for Development in Vienna. Research strategies were subsumed by these broader agendas.

In the early 1980s, the need for a WHO research strategy to match the health-for-all strategy became more pressing. Consequently, the Director-General appointed Prof. T. McKeown to chair a subcommittee of the ACMR on health research strategy (1983–88). The subcommittee's report (8) was discussed by the governing bodies at global as well as regional levels (1986-88) and came to the conclusion that achieving health for all was to be defined more precisely as a level of health below which it was hoped that no country would fall – i.e. infant mortality below 50 (per 1000 live births) and life expectancy at birth of 60 years. It was recalled that these levels were reached in the middle of the 20th century by developed countries and more recently in some developing countries.

The determinants of the global health picture were also described and the consequential approaches to research planning were discussed, based on the following key observations (*11*) (WHO/RPD/ACHR (HRS) 86) and ACHR 29/88.5):

The human genetic constitution was much the same today as it was a hundred thousand years ago. That is to say, we now face vastly changed conditions of life with the same genetic equipment of our ancestors who were hunter-gatherers.

The modern transformation of health in the developed countries and the associated increase of populations, which began more than a century before effective medical intervention was possible, was to be attributed largely to improvements in living conditions.

Research had shown us the nature of infectious disease and the possibility of its prevention by environmental measures and immunization.

It had been recognized in the last few decades that most noncommunicable diseases could be prevented by changes in living conditions and behaviour; the most striking evidence being the recent decline of coronary deaths.

In 1986 it was considered that countries with very limited resources should give higher priority to research and services in nutrition, immunization and sanitation.

In order to further elaborate the formulation of a WHO research strategy, and following the technical discussions on "research for health for all" held at the Forty-third World Health Assembly in 1990, the ACHR drew on the work of its own subgroups, namely the task forces on science and technology, on health development research, and on "evolving problems of critical significance to health", and the subcommittees on health and the economy and on research capability strengthening.

The ACHR considered that although the health research strategy adopted in 1988 was still a valid cornerstone of WHO's research strategy, new dimensions should be added to give proper emphasis to infrastructural, economic, environmental and behavioural aspects. The revised strategy (9) focused on: the relevance of health and the economy, global problems and solutions, health research and human development, science and technology policies, the emergence of new ethical issues, and the strengthening of research capability in developing countries. It further emphasized key observations: a world in transition, the changing scene of science and technology, and the importance of identifying research needs on the basis of health needs. In 1993, the ACHR issued its report on *Research for health: principles, perspectives and strategies* (WHO/RPD/ACHR [HRS] 93).

In the following years, the ACHR attempted to further develop and refine the strategic approach, publishing in 1998 its *Research policy agenda for science and technology to support global health development* (19). The document emphasized that:

- there is a common fate, condition and ethic of all humanity that unifies action for global health development;
- while most health impacts are local, many underlying causes and potential solutions are global and multifactorial in nature;
- global health challenges, problems and determinants call for a more systematic global approach in support of action at international, national and local levels;
- the world's scientists and scientific institutions must work together and with all relevant partners, not only in conventional biomedical research but in all research that contributes to health;
- "intelligent" research networks need to be expanded or developed around major issues, taking advantage of appropriate communication technologies;
- a continuous process for definition, planning, implementation and evaluation of global research imperatives and opportunities is required.

It also proposed some novel methodological approaches for the graphic spatio-temporal description of health profiles (see Figure 2).

FIG. 2   **Tunisia's visual health information profile for 1994 (outlined in white) superimposed on that for 1966**

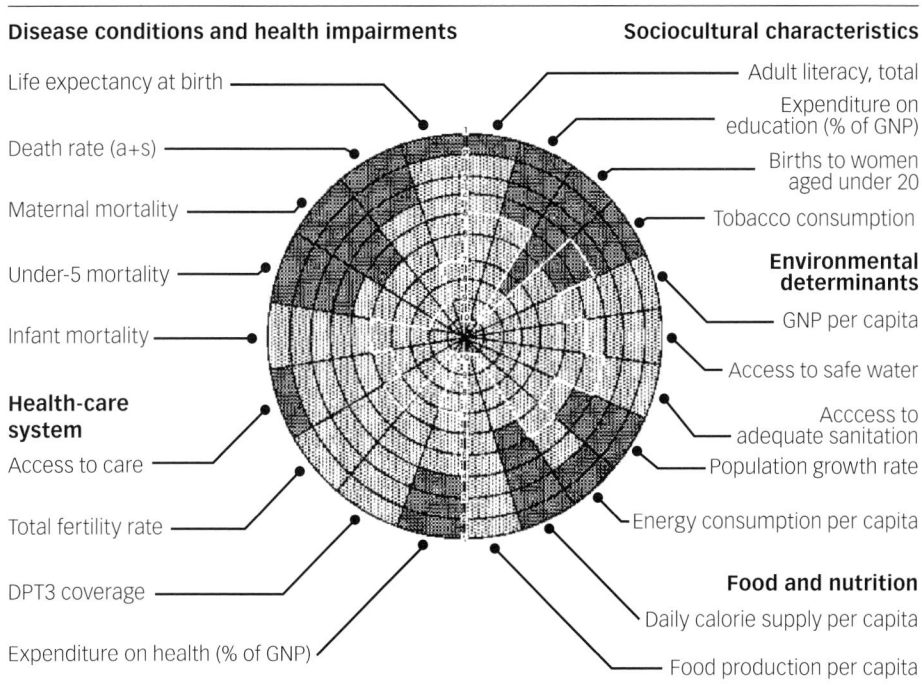

Source: Bulletin of the World Health Organization, 1999, 77(2) (http://www.who.int/bulletin/archives/77(2)176.pdf).

4. Research structures and processes: the means to an end

4.1 Documenting disparities in research

The 90/10 gap concept was well documented by the United Nations Office of Science and Technology in the 1970s in preparation for the UN Conference on Science and Technology for Development in 1979 and thereafter (5). Such documentation shows that the disparities in research arising from socioeconomic stresses can be summarized readily (see Table 3 a–b, and c–d).

3c and 3d reproduced from: *The role of health research in the strategy for Health for All by the year 2000*, which was used as background for technical discussions held during the World Health Assembly in May 1990 (22). Data cited do not necessarily agree with current WHO estimates for the years given.

A chapter was devoted to this issue in the WHO background paper submitted to the technical discussions held during the World Health Assembly in 1990. The concept of the 90/10 gap would later be extended to stress the imbalance in resource allocation between the South (10% of resources for those who suffer 90% of the disease burden) and the North (90% of resources for those with 10% of the disease burden).

In general, there was a growing recognition of the importance of financing research and development (R&D) activities in developing countries, and many countries in the past attempted to reach a minimum target of R&D expenditure at 0.5% of GNP. In 1985, all developing countries together reached an expenditure of US$ 14.3 billion or 0.66% of their GNP. In the same year, worldwide expenditure on R&D was US$ 330 billion dollars, according to United Nations estimates. The 1985 data show, however, that in a substantially large number of developing countries the allocation for R&D was far below the suggested level of 0.5% of GNP. In many countries, even where this target was met, the volume of funds was far below real needs because of the low levels of GNP.

The deleterious effects on the funding of R&D that were due to insignificant and sometimes negative growth rates of GNP were compounded by the effects of high inflation and the external debt crisis. The progress in the average level of funding of R&D in developing countries from 0.36% of GNP in 1973 to 0.66% of GNP in 1985 masks the fact that only 21 out of 124 developing countries accounted for nearly 95% of the R&D expenditures of all of them together.

Of these estimates of R&D funding, the proportion that went to health research was on average 10%, while research in agriculture and manufacturing received a much higher level of support.

To a large extent, the sources of the external funds for science and technology for development consisted of the developed countries and the international organizations

TABLE 3. **Disparities in research expenditure between countries according to economic status**

3a Distribution of population and resources between North and South (approximations)

	NORTH (%)	SOUTH (%)
Gross national product	80	20
Research and development	95	5
Scientists and engineers	90	10
Population	20	80

3b Research and development resources and production: North vs. South

		DEVELOPED (EME + FSE)	DEVELOPING	DIFFERENTIAL (PER CAPITA)
In	US$	450 billion	25 billion	100:1
	Scientists and engineers	4.3 million	0.6 million (China) + 0.7 million (all others)	7:1 25:1
	Publications	90%	10%	50:1
	Patents	99%	1%	500:1

Sources: World science report (UNESCO, 1996) and WHO data (from presentation at PAHO/ACHR/97.11 by B. Mansourian). EME: Established market economies. FSE: Former Soviet economies.

3c Estimated relative percentage expenditure on research and development in different sectors by country groups

COUNTRY GROUPS	AGRICULTURE	MANUFACTURING INDUSTRIAL	NON-MANUFACTURING INDUSTRIAL	HEALTH	ALL OTHER	TOTAL
All developing	29	39	3	10	19	100
Low-income	63	7	2	9	19	100
Middle-income	23	47	3	9	17	100
Capital surplus oil exporting	14	21	13	17	35	100
OECD less industrialized	20	38	5	7	30	100
OECD more industrialized	4	58	4	6	28	100

3d Central government expenditure on health (as % of total expenditure)

	1972	1987
Low-income countries (other than China and India)	5.4	3.4
China	–	–
India	1.5	1.9
Middle-income economies	6.3	5.1
Lower middle-income economies	5.8	3.5
Upper middle-income economies	6.7	–
Highly indebted countries	8.4	5.9

within and outside the United Nations system. A small portion was derived, during the 1970s and 1980s, from voluntary private funding organizations.

4.2 Principles of scientific cooperation for WHO

The original mechanisms utilized by WHO for scientific cooperation were summarized in a lecture presented at a meeting of the American Association for the Advancement of Science (AAAS) in Washington, DC, in 1972 by M. Kaplan (23). In that lecture, Dr Kaplan told his audience: "Collaborative research is the principal approach used in the WHO programme. This approach is based on the premise that certain problems are best attacked through cooperative efforts of workers in various countries operating under different ecological conditions".[1]

At that time, WHO had developed a network of some 750 reference centres and collaborating laboratories. As a rule, research projects were initiated and designed by technical units in WHO aided by consultants. The research itself was usually carried out by established institutions, including the above network of laboratories, often with modest financial assistance by WHO in the form of 'seed' grants to offset partially the much greater expenses borne by the laboratories themselves. The major element in successes that were achieved, according to Kaplan, lay in the goodwill, talent, and resources of collaborating scientists and their laboratories and institutes to which WHO had ready access. These research institutes were found worldwide in government services, universities and sometimes in commercial enterprises.

Small grants were also made by WHO to individual investigators working on subjects of interest to the organization, for training in research methodology, as well as to finance visits to other laboratories by scientists working on problems of mutual interest. When scientists bid for these grants, the applications were examined by technical units at WHO in consultation with outside referees, and by a special WHO grants committee. (At that time WHO also awarded more than 3500 education and training fellowships each year.)

---

[1] As at December 1972, the following results were claimed:
  (1) Evaluation of the effectiveness, or lack thereof, of recently developed biological products (vaccines and serums) for polio, measles, smallpox, rabies, typhoid, cholera, tuberculosis, brucellosis, leptospirosis, and cysticercosis.
  (2) Clarification of the epidemiology of the above group of diseases as well as of cancer, cardiovascular diseases, influenza, dengue and other parasitic diseases including malaria, toxoplasmosis, schistosomiasis, and hydatidosis among others.
  (3) Characterization of immune-complex nephritis in malaria and shock syndrome in dengue hemorrhagic fever.
  (4) Comparative studies in the chemotherapy of yaws, tuberculosis, leprosy, schistosomiasis, and brucellosis.
  (5) Insights into malnutrition, especially protein-calorie deficiencies and their relationship to infective agents.
  (6) Studies on the biology of many insect vectors and of their resistance to insecticides.
  (7) The development of nearly 300 biological standards and working preparations to provide baseline references for all countries.
  (8) Progress in international uniformity of diagnostic criteria and technical procedures for many of the major communicable and noncommunicable diseases (such as malnutrition, mental disorders, and the chronic degenerative diseases).

Apart from the AMCR, Kaplan explained, WHO periodically convened groups of experts to review specific subjects from a purely scientific point of view, to identify gaps in knowledge, to recommend research approaches, and to establish technical principles and guides. Members of these groups were drawn from 44 expert advisory panels totalling more than 2600 scientists appointed by the Director-General.

The International Agency for Research on Cancer (IARC) was formed as an autonomous body within WHO in 1965 to promote international collaboration in cancer research. The agency had (and still has) a governing council and a scientific advisory body. It operated at that time on an annual budget of about US$ 2.5 million from contributions of 10 participating countries. Located in Lyon, France, and working in close collaboration with WHO headquarters in Geneva, IARC concentrated on epidemiological investigations in many parts of the world and on laboratory research in Lyon.

WHO headquarters also carried out direct research in fields such as epidemiology and communication sciences. In addition, scientists were employed in WHO and its regional offices to work in institutions largely financed from sources external to the regular budget of WHO. In the 1970s, these include the Institute of Nutrition of Central America and Panama, the Pan American Zoonoses Centre near Buenos Aires, Argentina, the East African Virus Research Institute in Entebbe, Uganda, and some of the WHO research and training centres for immunology.

4.3 WHO mechanisms for the acquisition of scientific and technical/technological advice

4.3.1 Background

There are informal and formal mechanisms for scientific and technical consultation in WHO. At the informal level, various groups and non-statutory bodies are being used, ranging from informal consultations to more structured advisory committees. At the formal level, the relevant mechanisms are subject to regulatory control by the WHO governing bodies as in the case of expert advisory panels and the advisory structures established in connection with the special programmes. Two more sources of expert advice should be mentioned: the WHO collaborating centres, and the nongovernmental organizations (NGO) in official relations with WHO.

4.3.2 WHO collaborating centres

The idea of using national institutions for international purposes dates back to the days of the League of Nations, when national laboratories were first designated as reference centres for the standardization of biological products. As soon as WHO was established, it appointed more reference centres, starting in 1947 with the World Influenza Centre in London for worldwide epidemiological surveillance.

As early as 1949, the second World Health Assembly laid down the policy (which has been followed since) that WHO should not establish international research institutions under its own auspices but that "research in the field of health is best advanced by assisting, coordinating and making use of the activities of existing institutions".

All WHO collaborating centres, whether they deal with research or not (most of them do), have been designated under this policy, which has undoubtedly enhanced national participation in the Organization's activities. There is, however, an exception to that policy, in the WHO Region of the Americas, where a number of "international health centres" – some with regional (hemisphere-wide functions and others with subregional functions – have been set up and are financed and administered by the Pan American Health Organization, the regional organization of WHO for the Americas.

A WHO collaborating centre is an institution designated by the Director-General of WHO to form part of an inter-institutional collaborative network set up by WHO in support of its programme at the country, intercountry, regional, interregional and global levels, as appropriate. But there is more to it than that. In line with the WHO policy and strategy of technical cooperation, a WHO collaborating centre must also participate in the strengthening of country resources, in terms of information, services, research and training, in support of national health development.

Designation is made with the agreement of the head of the establishment to which the institution is attached or with that of the director of the institution, if it is independent, and after consultation with the national government. An institution is designated initially for a term of four years; the designation may be renewed for the same or a shorter period.

Those not eligible for designation (as initially intended for WHO collaborating centres) are, for example, networks, working groups, partnerships and programmes, or NGOs and similar bodies with a membership structure, including professional associations or foundations.

4.3.3 Functions and role of WHO collaborating centres

The functions of the WHO collaborating centres are manifold, and may include the following:

- collection, collation and dissemination of information;
- standardization of terminology and nomenclature, of technology, of diagnostic, therapeutic and prophylactic substances, and of methods and procedures;
- development and application of appropriate technology;
- provision of reference substances and other services;
- participation in collaborative research developed under the Organization's leadership, including the planning, conduct, monitoring and evaluation of research, as well as promotion of the application of the results of research;
- training, including research training;
- the coordination of activities carried out by several institutions on a given subject.

The main role of the WHO collaborating centres was to provide strategic support to the organization to meet two main needs:

1. Implementing WHO's mandated work and programme objectives
2. Developing and strengthening institutional capacity in countries and regions.

The WHO collaborating centres are an essential and cost-effective cooperation mechanism, which enables the organization to fulfil its mandated activities and to harness resources far exceeding its own. WHO gains access to top centres worldwide and the institutional capacity to ensure the scientific validity of global health work. Through these global networks, the organization is able to exercise leadership in shaping the international health agenda. Conversely, designation as a WHO collaborating centre provides institutions with enhanced visibility and recognition by national authorities, calling public attention to the health issues on which they work. It opens up improved opportunities for them to exchange information and develop technical cooperation with other institutions, in particular at international level, and to mobilize additional and sometimes important resources from funding partners.

A detailed analytical study was carried out by Professor M. Manciaux under the auspices of the ACHR in 1998 (see *24*).

4.3.4 *Pan American Health Organization centres*

By the 1970s the Pan American Health Organization (PAHO) had developed a complex network of centres of various types, which were instrumental in the development of WHO's programme in the Region of the Americas.

Ten PAHO centres were set up as international institutions administered by PAHO itself: seven of these centres were "hemisphere-wide" and three were of more limited subregional scope. The centres were located in eight different countries of the region and dealt with subjects that included disease prevention and control, nutrition, environmental health, maternal and child health, the teaching of biomedical technology, biomedical information, and the impact on health of economic and industrial development.

PAHO also enlisted the cooperation of associated national centres of three types:

> Type I: a national centre with some international involvement (e.g. the Training Centre in Immunology, Mexico);
> Type II: a national centre carrying out a substantial international function (e.g. the Research and Training Centre for Leprosy and Tropical Diseases, Caracas);
> Type III: a centre performing an international function, including service to the host country, essentially similar to PAHO centres (e.g. the Research and Reference Centre on Vector Biology and Control, Maracay).

The report of a committee chaired by Prof. M. Wegman (*25*) submitted to the Pan American Sanitary Conference/WHO Regional Committee for the Americas in 1978, concluded that "the existing centres are performing useful and important services and help significantly in fulfilling PAHO's mission".

Finally, it stated that "adapting a national centre to a broader international role by a cooperative arrangement" whether through a Pan American or an associated national centre, is "a way for a country to share its expertise abroad" and "an effective illustration of the concept of technical cooperation among developing countries".

4.4 Research capacity strengthening and the special programmes

Strengthening the scientific and technological infrastructure is part and parcel of WHO's mandate to promote health-related research. Formal concerns about this issue were expressed by WHO's management, as well as by the ACMR and the governing bodies in the early and mid-1970s. This led, *inter alia*, to the creation of TDR and the fostering of the "special programme" approach. It also led to setting up the five regional ACMRs (PAHO having had its own since 1962), supported by specific secretariats.

These efforts were aimed at supporting national self-relevance in health-related research, as appeared clearly from the several consultations, symposia, workshops initiated throughout the 1980s, by regional and national organizers. For the last quarter of the 20th century, the discourse and related actions focused on methods for developing infrastructures (management, training, information, career structures, special programme support etc). A number of issues that have occupied major discussion fora in the scientific community, especially in relation to essential national research, are described below.

4.4.1 Infrastructural and managerial problems

Although considerable progress has been made in development of infrastructure for health research in developing countries, the overall picture is not satisfactory. For example, during the 1970s and 1980s, little more than half of member countries in the African Region had medical research councils or analogous bodies and fewer still had developed a national health research policy and priorities in support of the health-for-all strategy. The situation in the developing countries in the Americas, Eastern Mediterranean, South East Asian and Western Pacific regions was somewhat better but left room for substantial improvement. WHO's goals stated that (i) at policy level, all countries should have a national health research policy including an appropriate decision-making process and that (ii) at management level, all countries should have established and/or strengthened their health research management and coordinating mechanisms including programme planning monitoring and evaluation, through the establishment of resources, policy management and coordination bodies such as medical/health research councils or analogous bodies.

In some disciplines, there was a need for specialized research institutions. Competent research workers and adequate research career structures were deemed necessary in all countries. Special programmes have regularly been subjected to external evaluations by independent high-level bodies.

4.4.2 Prioritizing action research

As the movement towards decentralization set in motion in the mid-1970s, the ACMR emphasized a number of principles. For instance, WHO Member States should participate in formulating national health research policies and in defining health research priorities (linked to solving pressing health problems), strategies and plans consistent with their development needs and goals. Scientific and technological infrastructure (including research manpower) would need to be strengthened and brought in line with

the national strategy. The cornerstone of any national health research effort, the ACHR stated, should be a coherent policy that would:
— identify health research priorities and problems, through valid epidemiological research;
— promote application of existing knowledge and technology to solve pressing health problems;
— encourage targeted or strategic research to obtain new tools for promotion of health and control of disease;
— permit a rational allocation of resources, however limited they may be;
— support sustained work towards clearly defined objectives, including especially the development of health research manpower and other research infrastructure, and mechanisms for research coordination and management.

In countries where the credibility of research as an essential tool for informed decision-making had yet to be established and the availability of financial and material resources for research was limited, the ACHR felt that research priorities could justifiably be focused on health systems or essential health research, field and community-based studies, improvement of existing evaluation procedures and establishment of a simple and reliable basic health information system. In the area of health systems research directed primarily towards the achievement of health for all through primary health care, the ACHR felt that research should provide managers and decision-makers at all levels with the information needed to make better decisions in solving health problems. Equally important was the need to involve health system managers and decision-makers in the determination of research priorities and the generation of research questions. To achieve this objective, it was recommended, flexible institutional linkages should be developed between decision-making in health and other health-related sectors (such as education, agriculture, etc.) and researchers in universities and scientific institutions.

An adequate and responsive information system was seen as a sine qua non for research and for utilization of research results. Highest priority needs to be given to the development of national capability, members of the ACHR said, to survey and keep up-to-date with available scientific knowledge to identify knowledge of potential importance to the country, to interpret and communicate it to policy-makers and decision-makers and to devise, organize, manage and evaluate studies to explore its applicability and effectiveness.

4.4.3 *Mechanisms for research capacity strengthening*
Elaborating on the previous points and with a view to the technical discussions on research at the World Health Assembly in 1990, the ACHR argued that research capacity strengthening (RCS) in developing countries should be considered as an integral part of national development. For example, while it may be necessary to carry out laboratory work aimed at developing new vaccines and drugs predominantly in developed countries, it is essential that the new products be assessed both in patients and communities in the endemic areas. Such assessment and transfer of research results would be best done by a core of competent "local" research workers well acquainted with local eco-

nomic, social and cultural circumstances as well as with the ecology, epidemiology and disease patterns of the countries, according to the ACHR. Moreover, it is essential that epidemiological, social and economic research be carried out in places in which the diseases under study are indigenous. In addition, if the WHO's special programmes such as TDR and HRP were to be efficient and not to continue indefinitely, it would be essential to build up research expertise and scientific institutions, appropriately funded in the developing countries.

The ACHR noted that where and when research institutions have been strengthened or created and researchers trained, the willingness of governments to provide long-term and continuous support was critical for sustained and adequate performance. It was equally important to develop and sustain a culture of national investment in basic, scientific and numerate education at all levels of learning, to attach high social status to science and technology and to evolve a tradition of research to solve problems. Ideally, research capability strengthening from external (bilateral, multilateral) assistance needs to be backed by national commitment as typified, ACHR pointed out, by the success stories of some institutions in Brazil, Cuba, Kenya, Malaysia, Papua New Guinea, Peru, Sri Lanka and Thailand.

A crucial aspect for long-term effectiveness of institutional strengthening is the commitment of governments to cover the recurrent cost of institutions after the external support has ceased. Such commitment is not always forthcoming. The experience of the WHO from its special and other programmes showed that RCS, though a long drawn-out process, could be achieved through a number of mechanisms. These included support in terms of research equipment, funds and training of personnel for selected institutions for 5 to 10 years, collaborative research and linkage of institutions in developing and developed countries, as well as linkage with developed countries, training, including group training of suitable personnel within and outside their countries, either short-term (e.g. workshops, symposia) or long-term (MSc, PhD training), provision of re-entry grants (to help trainees establish their lines of work in home institutions) and visiting scientist grants for established scientists to visit both developed and developing countries.

The ACHR concluded that it is important that young trained researchers be carefully nurtured and encouraged within a well articulated research manpower training plan and manpower development policy. Every country should recognize and address the issues related to health research career structure – the need for it, adaptation to national priorities, the desirable incentives, and the resources and constraints involved, the goal being to increase national capability to conduct research and to prevent brain drain.

4.4.4 Developing networks

Linkages to foster collaboration in research and research manpower training provide an effective means of developing RCS and reducing the sense of isolation experienced by scientists in developing countries. Such linkages have brought together research institutions in developed countries with those in developing countries, or have connected groups of research institutions in developing countries who share common health problems but at varying levels of infrastructure or needs. In one of its meetings leading up to the technical discussions at the World Health Assembly in 1990, the ACHR cited examples of successful linkages between the Institute of Public Health in Manila with the Walter and Eliza Hall Institute of Medical Research in Melbourne, and between the Kenya Institute of Medical Research and institutions in the USA. The ACHR pointed out that, with health research becoming increasingly multidisciplinary and multisectoral, it is important for researchers to establish links with their peers from other disciplines and institutions.

4.4.5 Research career structures

No health research can succeed without the human resources or "brain ware" to implement it. The creation of an attractive research career structure in developing countries contributes a crucial component of RCS and a long-term research strategy; yet it is a task which has been neglected by most developing countries, in spite of repeated emphasis by the WHO, and the Global and Regional Advisory Committees on Health Research. The recruitment, training and the subsequent productive employment of talented nationals in the countries' health research programmes is a decisive factor for the long-term success of their research efforts. It is important to stress that promotion of a research career structure is not an end in itself, but the means to support research activities as a basic component of health policies, strategies and plans. The success of the development of a research career structure is very much dependent on its synchronization with overall institution strengthening in research. Professional satisfaction, stemming from the availability of adequate means to carry out research is as important as remuneration and other benefits for the serious and dedicated research worker. Lack of such professional satisfaction is a major cause of "brain drain" from the research field to other areas within countries or to work outside the countries. While equitable salaries are necessary, the non-monetary incentives are equally desirable. Research disciplines which are important but possibly unattractive to young people might be designated "hardship areas" – and receive special attention and allowances.

4.4.6 UNDP/World Bank/WHO Special Programme for Research and Training in Tropical Diseases: research capability strengthening[1]

The reorganization of TDR's components (operational units) in 1987 focused primarily on the programme's efforts to strengthen the research capability of developing endemic countries. The objectives set at that time for TDR's Research Capability Strengthening Component were:

— to integrate the programme's activities in research capability strengthening and in research and development;
— to identify the institutions and research workers in developing countries that could make the best use of support to further the research and development objectives of the programme;

---

[1] A comprehensive overview of the first 30 years of TDR was published in 2007. See further reading.

BOX 9

New policies and structures for the Special Programme for Research and Training in Tropical Diseases, 1987

Policies and structures for TDR in 1987

New policies

TDR's new policies for research capability strengthening permeate all areas of work. Research and development is used increasingly to promote research capability strengthening objectives (for the training of and research by scientists in tropical disease-endemic countries). In practice, this policy change has resulted in closer working relations between the Steering Committees for Research and Development Components and the Research Strengthening Group, which manages research capability strengthening. They work together, for example, to select potential recipients of support among institutions and scientists in developing endemic countries, to monitor the progress that recipients of assistance have made in their capability to conduct research and in their scientific output, to organize group training in workshops, seminars and the like , and to identify suitable research projects (especially field trials of disease-control tools) for "hands-on" training of scientists in developing countries. The change in policy has also introduced an element of competitiveness among applicants for grants for institution-strengthening and research training.

Greater emphasis is being placed on human, as against material, resources. A comprehensive system of funding can provide support for a scientist at all stages of a scientific career. But again the focus is on scientific productivity, not on training for the sake of training. The training itself is increasingly geared to local disease-control requirements and involves more community-based research, notably field research, which includes epidemiological, entomological, and social and economical studies.

Linkages and networking have also been introduced to a greater degree in virtually all mechanisms for strengthening research capability. A number of new grants provide for linkages between institutions and scientists in industrialized and developing countries, and the longer-established grants emphasize collaboration between those in different countries within a region or in different regions. The aim is to make the most effective use of the programme's support by helping to establish a worldwide network of skills and talents in diverse and complementary disciplines. North-South linkages, in particular, should promote the exchange of resources between, on the one hand, research workers in industrialized countries with an abundance of technological facilities but little contact with tropical field conditions and, on the other, scientists in developing countries who could apply this technology to improved control of tropical diseases.

Finally, a differential approach is being introduced into research capability strengthening policy. Research groups or scientists in developing countries who have reasonably well developed research resources and well established research training programmes are being encouraged to apply for institution-strengthening grants, awarded on a competitive basis. By contrast, in areas lacking such resources or training facilities, the programme relies more for research capability strengthening on setting up field research projects within, wherever possible, the national government's disease-control programmes. For administrative purposes, grants awarded under the research capability strengthening programme fall into two main groups: institution-strengthening grants and research training grants. For practical purposes, though, they are interlinked. Research training requires adequate research facilities, which may need strengthening. Similarly, strengthening an

> institution so that it can fully participate in a research partnership often calls for support for its training facilities and for the training of its staff.
>
> **New structures**
> Field research is a high priority: it is the critical link between biotechnology and disease control. Field Links for Intervention and Control Studies (FIELDLINKS) is a recently created programme deigned to promote high quality field research on the TDR diseases (malaria, schistosomiasis, filariasis, try-panosomiasis, leishmaniasis and leprosy). The goal of the FIELDLINKS programme is to stimulate and support field research which will lead to improved control strategies for tropical diseases.
>
> The three objectives of the programme are: (1) to provide training in epidemiology, entomology and social sciences for individuals conducting field research on intervention strategies and implementing control programmes, (2) to promote field research networks as mechanisms for training in project design, methodologies and techniques of field research, and for project linkage which will reduce the isolation of investigators; and (3) to work in close collaboration with TDR's disease-specific components to provide input into the selection and utilization of epidemiological, social science and entomological methods appropriate for the study of tropical diseases.
>
> In 1987 an Initiative for Biotechnology Implementation was launched, partly in fulfilment of TDR's mandate to promote the application and transfer of advances in biomedical sciences to tropical disease research and control and partly to fill a need for the local production in the endemic countries of biotechnology tools used in field research projects and national disease control programmes. The initiative covered specific projects for the production of key reagents in sufficient quantities and in suitable formulations for cost-effective use in the producing countries. The reagents included monoclonal antibodies, recombinant-derived and synthetic antigens, and nucleic acid probes that will be used for the diagnosis of infection and disease, parasite identification and characterization, and the evaluation of candidate vaccines, as well as in epidemiological studies on disease transmission and vector control.
>
> Other initiatives included the provision of research training, postgraduate field research training, career development and institution strengthening grants.

— to strengthen links between institutions, research projects and national disease-control programmes in the developing countries in which the target diseases are endemic;
— to focus on obtaining concrete scientific results from strengthening the research capability of persons and institutions.

New policies and new structures were introduced in 1987 and are described in Box 9.

4.4.7 WHO Special Programme of Research, Development and Research Training in Human Reproduction: strengthening national research capabilities in human reproduction

Twenty years after its inception, the Special Programme on Research, Development and Research Training in Human Reproduction (HRP) was spending a third of its operational budget on strengthening the research capacities of developing countries. The purpose was to assist these countries to carry out research to solve problems in reproductive health, which includes fertility regulation. Many developing countries required assistance in accurately defining their reproductive health problems and in drawing up a realistic research agenda. The special programme, working with research institutions and ministries of health in these countries, helped these institutions to formulate five-year research development plans and also supported the implementation of these plans although, during the first 20 years of HRP, restrictions on resources limited such activities to 26 developing countries, including the training of nearly 600 researchers.

Since the commencement of HRP in 1972 and until 1986, RCS activities were largely focused on developing institutional capacities to assist them collaborate in multicentre research initiated by the special programme. After 1986, the direction of RCS activities turned towards meeting national research needs in reproductive health. The change of direction was reflected in the strategic plan that was first developed in 1986 for the purpose of strengthening research capabilities of developing countries.

The policies described in the 1986 strategic plan emphasized the need for countries to formulate national strategic plans for reproductive health research based on an assessment of research needs. HRP's support for RCS in countries was time-limited and in the case of any single institution would normally not exceed 10 years. As special programme support was phased out over an agreed period of time, national authorities were expected gradually to take over recurrent expenditures within their national budgets and thus help to institutionalize health research in their respective national development activities. The development of research manpower was a major aspect of these strengthening activities; for this purpose HRP had in its first 20 years provided over 1000 training grants to staff of research institutions in developing countries and, where appropriate, assisted in setting up research career structures.

By the early 1990s, HRP described its mission as to promote the development of a global network of institutions capable of carrying out research and research training as related to reproductive health including fertility regulation. Such a network could be possible only if there were competent research workers in well-equipped and well-managed research institutions in developing countries. The special programme's role was to promote and support what were essentially national and institutional efforts. Nevertheless, with a broad vision of the target for a global network of nationally-supported institutions engaged in high-quality research and research training in all aspects or human reproduction, HRP proposed to focus on the achievement of a range of objectives at institutional, national and regional levels (see Box 10).

HRP outlined specific strategies for the strengthening of research capacities to match the stage of research development in the respective countries. For instance:

BOX 10

Objectives of the Special Programme on Research, Development and Research Training in Human Reproduction after 1986

HRP objectives after 1986: strengthening national research capabilities

In institutions
— A critical mass of researchers competent in the basic biological, pharmacological, clinical, epidemiological, biostatistical and social sciences, performing quality research of national relevance and of scientific importance;

— Scientific leadership and managerial competence, in all supported institutions;

— Educationally-sound programmes of training for research related to reproductive health including fertility regulation;

— Strong linkages with national family-planning programmes;

— Strong national support for the institution's research and training activities, as demonstrated by the creation of suitable research career structures and by progressive increase in the national funding of research into reproductive health including fertility regulation;

— Well-maintained physical and laboratory facilities for the investigations required for research into reproductive health including fertility regulation and also facilities for the processing of data;

— A research review mechanism to assess productivity and to evaluate and disseminate research results;

— A mechanism for the regular review of progress in training programmes and in development of the total institution; and

— A mechanism for peer review of proposed research and to ensure ethical standards.

In each country
— An efficient system of organization for the national coordination of research in reproductive health including fertility regulation, to ensure that research is not unnecessarily duplicated, that research and evaluation results are translated into practice, that local resources are efficiently coordinated, and that local research corresponds with the national definition of research needs and priorities;

— A close collaboration between the family health service systems and the research institutions;

— Increasing national support for research and research training related to all aspects of fertility regulation; and

— A national forum for the research workers where they can present and discuss their results with programme personnel, policy-makers and administration.

In each region
In the regions, research strategies must take into account the political constraints that make collaborative programmes difficult, but provide for the maximum exchange of experience and information within and between the regions. The Special Programme will aim at achieving the following targets:

Continued page 42

> — Collaborative research programmes between neighbouring countries with similar problems, especially problems concerning access to fertility regulation services;
> — Centre of special expertise that plays a regional role especially for research training in the different academic disciplines required for research in reproductive health, including the social sciences; and
> — Active collaboration in research and in institutional development activities among institutions engaged in Special Programme-supported programmes.
>
> The Special Programme is willing to support national and local research, particularly, in those countries whose governments have committed themselves to assume phased responsibility for supporting the research. However, it must be recognized that not all governments do so. Some that do not yet recognize the need for research policies of family planning services may do so once research findings demonstrate the need. Such countries should not be categorically excluded from efforts to strengthen research capability, nor are those countries which may have the interest but lack the economic resources to absorb support for research institutions. Support should go to the kind of research that a country is likely to support in the long term.

- **Countries with minimal research activities:**
  Universities were being recognized as nonexclusive focal points for efforts to develop institutions. HRP aimed to identify promising individuals with potential for scientific leadership, wherever they were located in the country, and support the development of research capability around them. That support would be mainly from staff development with a view to creating a critical mass of research workers. Wherever possible, the more developed institutions in the special programme network were to be offered the opportunity of training these individuals.

- **Countries with a moderate amount of ongoing research activities:**
  The first step was normally to identify the most suitable institution, in consultation with the national government in accordance with the country's strategic plan from health research, and to offer a mix of support for training their staff and developing other research infrastructure. A substantial amount of consultant advice was provided on-site to assist in preparing good research protocols in the context of a long-term institutional development plan.

- **Countries with well developed research programmes:**
  Where research was well established, strengthening activities consisted mainly of helping scientists to apply for funds from research projects from HRP's task forces dealing with special areas of research and from other agencies. Here, HRP considered requests for support for staff training mainly to learn specific new investigative techniques and to keep in touch generally with advances in the field. The main concern of the special programme was to assist institutions to train scientists from less-developed institutions, and to maintain them as active units in the global institutional network.

4.5 Convening major stakeholders in global health

One of many examples of a gathering of major stakeholders is the meeting of the heads of collaborating centres (*26*) for a particular network. It is worth recalling that several times during ACHR meetings, Nobel Laureate Joshua Lederberg referred to the "convening power of WHO". Lederberg's contribution to scientific thinking within WHO can be illustrated by this quotation from 1998:

> "The ravaging epidemic of acquired immunodeficiency syndrome has shocked the world. It is still not comprehended widely that it is a natural, almost predictable, phenomenon. We will face similar catastrophes again, and will be ever more confounded in dealing with them, if we do not come to grips with the realities of the place of our species in nature. A large measure of humanistic progress is dedicated to the subordination of human nature to our ideals of individual perfectibility and autonomy. Human intelligence, culture, and technology have left all other plant and animal species out of the competition. We also may legislate human behaviour. But we have too many illusions that we can, by writ, govern the remaining vital kingdoms, the microbes, that remain our competitors of last resort for dominion of the planet. The bacteria and viruses know nothing of national sovereignties. In that natural evolutionary competition, there is no guarantee that we will find ourselves the survivor" (*26*).

Throughout its first 50 years, WHO retained its two pillars: a normative function and technical cooperation. The former embodied long-term commitments such as international agreements on the classification of tumours and the *International classification of diseases and related health problems* (ICD), setting up food safety standards, and creating lists of essential drugs. WHO also fulfilled the role of an alert and response system at the onset of major global epidemics (e.g. AIDS, BSE, SARS, and H5N1).

WHO's decentralized structure has facilitated technical cooperation. This has allowed regional offices closer contact with Member States and faster technical interventions in the case of natural or manmade disasters. A classic example of worldwide cooperation is in monitoring the influenza virus.

5. The broad range of WHO's research activities

The following section refers to the very broad spectrum of research-related activities discussed, promoted and reviewed by the ACMR/ACHR system. It cites some 'forward-looking initiatives'. It elaborates on 'methodological' as well as 'substantive' themes which portray the scope of interest in all of WHO's work. It also reviews all the major initiatives related to 'Strategy Formulation' in the last quarter of the twentieth century.

5.1 Subjects discussed by the ACMR and ACHR

The range of issues tabled for the committee's overview and advice covered practically every aspect of WHO's work as demonstrated by the agendas of the years 1972–98.

5.2 Forward-looking initiatives in research

In the course of its history, WHO witnessed some original developments, briefly cited here.

5.2.1 Research in epidemiology and communication science

Dr. M. Candau, WHO's Director-General from 1953 to 1973, considered science and research as a core value in WHO's mission, and the "Plan for an Intensified Research Programme" coincided with his first years in office. The eventual outcome of the plan was no less than a "proposal for the establishment of a World Health Research Centre". However, given the lack of political support for a full-scale project, three distinct entities eventually came into being: the International Agency for Research on Cancer (IARC) in 1965, an international network for monitoring adverse reactions to drugs, and the WHO Division of Research in Epidemiology and Communication Sciences (RECS), both established in 1967. A relatively detailed account of the history of RECS is given in the WHO history series (3).

5.2.2 Early warning systems

In a communication to AAAS (December 1972), M. Kaplan (23) argued that there was a great need for a rapid development of a computerized health information network linking all countries to a centralized facility in Geneva. He predicted that it would take decades to achieve. Of special value, would be research in the mathematics of epidemiological theory (27), in technological assessment, in operations research (28), and in analytical techniques for extracting meaningful correlations from a large number of variables. The same paper pointed out to the need for "technological aids", including pattern recognition (*29,30*) and bio-instrumentation for diagnostic and survey procedures, as well as inexpensive technologies for coping with environmental pollutants, improving sanitation, and designing prosthetic devices. Specific projects had been encouraged in these domains (*31*, also see *Further reading*). Satellite-related technologies had been identified at an early stage too (see *Further reading*). Of special interest in respect of early warning systems was a consultation on the subject held at WHO headquarters, 31July–2 August 1974. The experts recommended the establishment of an "alert system" in WHO with the following aims:

— to establish a basic knowledge of the dynamic statistical properties within populations of health-status indicators selected with reference to the priorities which are established by WHO for an alerting system;
— to collect and validate all available data on the selected health-status indicators on an ongoing basis;
— to process these data by appropriate techniques so as to obtain evidence for or against the need to issue an alert;
— to extract from the data a measure of the statistical reliability of the judgement that is made.

5.2.3 Geographic information systems

The early 1980s saw the progressive adoption and expansion of personal computing in WHO. Although not a distinct outcome of the early warning system effort, the work on geographic information systems (GIS) was a logical forward-looking development (Figure 3). Drs. Nuttall and Mott pioneered the application of the methodology in WHO, initially in the areas of schistosomiasis and dracunculiasis (*32*). Dr. Nuttall subsequent-

FIG. 3 **Geographic information systems**

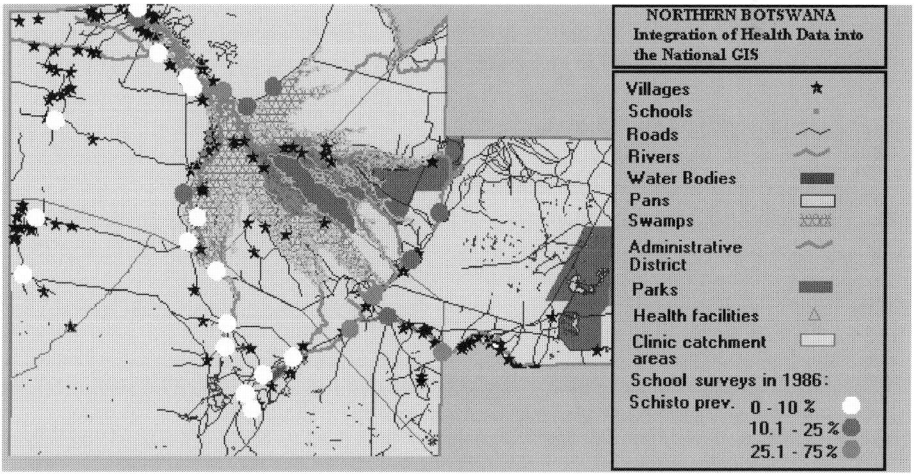

One of the first maps produced for WHO by Dr I Nuttall and the late Dr K Mott, using GIS (1993). The map shows an overlay of schistosomiasis survey data on national environmental information. Reproduced courtesy of Dr I Nuttall. Presented as an example only.

ly developed the work with other colleagues, applying GIS to African trypanosomiasis, lymphatic filariasis and malaria (33).

5.2.4 Pattern analysis

Methods derived from electrical engineering (including fast Fourier transforms, or FFT, and digital filtering) were utilized in WHO for the first time under the aegis of RECS, and the Office of Science and Technology. Prof. B. McA. Sayers summarized the approach in *Research methods for health development* (30).

When patterns exist in a health – or health-related – variable it can be assumed that underlying mechanisms of a systematic, as distinct from random, kind are operative. Pattern analysis therefore aims to identify characteristics of the variable that might offer useful indications about the nature of its generating mechanisms. The approach therefore needs techniques to indicate the presence of systematic structure in the data, methods for its selective enhancement, insight into the effects and consequences of the existence of the systematic structure, and a battery of methods to indicate likely mechanisms that could produce the systematic structure observed.

The earliest studies on an epidemiological time series in diarrhoeal disease, were published in 1975 (34). A subsequent application analysed the spatio-temporal patterns of a rabies epizootic in Europe (35). Further investigations have since developed internationally.

5.2.5 Systems analysis

The application of systems science in public health issues of interest to WHO has been periodically discussed, especially during the 1970s. The subject has also elicited academic investigations on global health, in collaboration with WHO (see Figure 4) (36).

A cogent discussion is to be found in the report of the ACMR Subcommittee on the Enhancement of Transfer of Technology to Developing Countries with Special Reference to Health, which referred to the "multisectoral structures that define the behaviour of communities, especially for health-care purposes". The subcommittee concluded that "health development planning in particular requires information about a number of interconnecting sectors that link with health.[1]

---

[1] The subcommittee's comments on systems analysis were as follows:

"Systems scientists deal with the identification, spontaneous behaviour and response to interventions, of self-contained assemblies of interconnecting components. These assemblies may take the form of physical or biological structures, or of behavioural, societal or economic elements. A chemical process plant is a typical industrial process system, which can be treated, in the first instance, as self-contained. The cardiovascular system is a well-defined physiological structure that can be treated as a system, though in this case of course, the system is subject to intervention and disturbance from other body systems. The interacting assembly of behavioural activities (or indeed of societal or economic activities) in a community also constitutes a system, although difficulties arise in identifying the elements, and the pathways and indeed the nature of their interconnections – that appears much more acutely in defining and studying the multisectoral structures that define the behaviour of communities, especially for health care purposes.

"The reason for approaching such structures in this way – defining the system and specifying its elements and their interconnections – is to achieve an improved understanding of both the spontaneous behaviour of the system and the nature of its responses to disturbances and interventions. To make possible the study

FIG. 4 Countries plotted according to their overall rank orders in socioeconomic and health dimensions for 1965

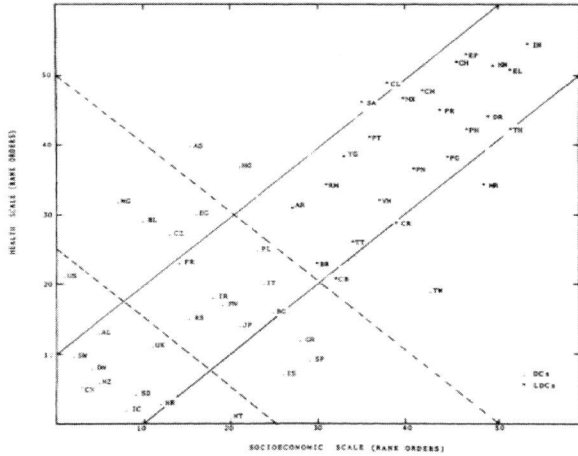

Note: The region between two solid lines represents balanced growth with respect to these two dimensions. Countries to the left of this region are "health inefficient", those to the right are "health efficient". Dashed lines separate most advanced countries from the remainder of developed and less developed countries. Reproduced as an example only.

---

of system behaviour it is necessary to model the system, identify the components and their interconnections, assign quantitative values to all pathways and finally simulate the system in some convenient way – say, in a computer model. Naturally all this can only be achieved on the basis of adequate measurement and interpretation of real data from the system to be studied: unavoidably a complex operation. Consequently various simplifying approaches may be taken, which are justified by expediency or by practicality. An example is the use of a static model, based on a path-analytic analysis; using a static model disregards the dynamics of the system altogether and sees the system only in terms of steady state conditions; path-analytic analysis disregards the complete feedback loop nature of most systems and deals only with static 'input-output' relations between defined variables thought to be related. Neither restriction is satisfactory as a final target, but is often helpful in the initial stages of an investigation. It is, however, commonly recognized that static models are very inadequate and may be highly misleading in important respects; the reason lies in the fact that disturbances (and no system can be imagined to be in a completely steady state),-or other changes that occurred at some unspecifiable time earlier-, take time to show their influence – and these disturbances may be unknown or unrecognized. In order to obtain a reasonably complete understanding of the system, its time-course behaviour – its dynamics – must therefore be taken into account. Fortunately there are well-defined techniques for studying the dynamics of complex systems; unfortunately these methods are themselves quite complicated and difficult to apply, especially in large-scale systems that involve human behaviour.

"One of the basic insights, applicable to all kinds of system, that has been reached, is that the structure of interconnections within a system is all important to its behaviour. Accordingly, the identification of the pattern and nature of interconnections within a system is critical to further analysis.

"A few words are warranted on the goals of system analysis. Descriptive models of a system can be computer-implemented and then subjected to test. Often the interest is in observing the consequences, and perhaps also the cost, of specific strategies of intervention designed to achieve some long-tern shift in the system. For instance, in a socioeconomic system involving societal, employment and health sectors, it may be a planner's intention to achieve some specific health-development target, for instance a shift in the mean level of some health variable such as the average weight of three-year-old infants; the target requires a strategy to obtain the resources needed – probably at the expense of other resource cost centres elsewhere in the system – and this strategy will have consequences and is optimum to achieve the target, in the light of the costs and consequences in other sectors. Naturally, advance information of this kind would be very useful to development planning of any kind, and health development planning in particular requires information about a number of interconnecting sectors that link with health; hence the health planner is unavoidably concerned with multisectoral systems and their behaviour: the form and nature of pathways and the dynamics of the intersectoral relations."

The subcommittee asserted that general systems theory has some helpful insights to offer to researchers. For instance, it recognizes that system boundaries are determined not only by objective reality but also by the questions that are to be asked about the system. It also recognizes that if the system has a significant degree of complexity, then full insight into the way the system behaves, and why, requires more than a single representation.[1]

---

[1] On the application of systems theory and new developments in modelling techniques, the subcommittee commented as follows:

The application of systems theory
"Both biological and social systems are 'open', self-regulating and adaptive. These systems behave as if goal-seeking and work through a 'hierarchy' of quasi-autonomous systems each of which has its own adaptive targets, the relative importance of which may alter continuously (in a physiological example, the muscular mechanics of the thoracic cage are not only involved in the physical effort of breathing, they are also concerned with posture and independent optimization probably occurs in respect of each function.)

By identifying features such as these, general systems theory is able to offer insights into the way to handle not only the complicated real systems that occur in technology but those that arise in biology, economics or social behaviour. General theory offers a framework of methodology by which to determine the components, linkages and parameters of any system (the process of identification) and by which to determine when adaptability, optimization, or goal-seeking, are operating and perhaps, to what purpose.

The general systems analysis approach also highlights several other features. For instance although systems analysis must begin with a drastically simplified version of the real system, the gap between reality and theory must always be remembered. It is a recognizable mistake to isolate one facet of the total problem, or one sector amongst several that interact. Oversimplifying the problem, or incorrectly simplifying it, does more damage than merely "getting the numbers wrong" – the whole system description may be hopelessly unrealistic. Specifically, in the analysis of complex systems, it is easy to neglect input and output components or systems parameters that turn out to be fundamentally important for the functioning of the system and for the understanding of its behaviour.

"It is also possible to identify other methodological problems in multisectoral modelling for instance: quantification of variables, quality of data, the need for a sufficient quantity of reliable data to allow for dynamic analysis, and the interpretation of the data as representing a determinant of say, health or of some other sector variable. How troublesome these are depends on the type of modelling being undertaken."

New developments in modelling techniques
"There are two fundamental difficulties about mathematical modelling – obtaining suitable data or making use of the data that can be obtained, and ensuring completeness. First, much of the relevant information about any socioeconomic system is non-quantitative, i.e. it cannot be expressed in numerical or algebraic terms. Second, the efficacy of the modelling may be grossly affected by the omission, from the model, of various pathways that exist within the real system – omitted because of the difficulty of measurement or because the existence of the specific pathway was not recognized. Some new technological approach is clearly needed to circumvent these difficulties. Developments in rule-based thinking are promising. The prospect is offered of utilizing qualitative information together with quantitative data about the system being studied. It should also, in principle, be easier to collect sufficient information about the real system to reduce the risk of missing significant system pathways. Furthermore, as explained below, the manner in which the analysis of input information is carried out should lead to a modelled system that is not strongly dependent on any a priori decisions about structure. The essence of the approach lies in the use of logic programming to analyse the logical relationships between inputs (so-called 'attributes') to, and outputs from the system under study and establish 'rules' which could, for instance, be used to forecast the 'output' when the attributes are specified. The 'rules' themselves are deduced by computer logic, using a logic-programming language, applied to a number of examples of the observed inputs and outputs drawn from the behaviour of the real system. There is no need for the data to be expressed in quantitative terms, qualitative statements about relevant aspects of the system are equally usable and may be much more realistic than quantitative data which can often only be obtained with difficulty and which would be frequently inappropriate in the description of the variable or indicator of interest. Further, there

5.2.6 Transfer of technology

The subject of transfer of technology was both transdisciplinary and transprogrammatic (a good example was the use of "expert systems" for vaccine production).

In 1983 the ACMR established a subcommittee under the chairmanship of Professor G.L. Ada to report, over a three-year period, on the "enhancement of transfer of technology to developing countries with special reference to health". This action was taken following discussion of a report by a working group on "the contribution of modern scientific concepts and methods to human health". The terms of reference (paraphrased) were:

- What health needs of developing countries can benefit from technology transfer?
- How can technology transfer from provider to user country be facilitated?
- What is the potential of the new ideas and technologies in the biological and physical sciences to contribute to better health?
- What can WHO do to help technology transfer?

As most of WHO's work is concerned with technology transfer, staff members from many programmes were interviewed; the subcommittee benefited greatly from such interactions.

The final report of the subcommittee was presented in October 1986 (*13*). It contained six annexes and three technical papers (see bibliography). The ACHR strongly endorsed the report and recommended that an executive version be prepared and circulated widely. Annex 1 contains a summary of the report's proposals.

5.3 Methodological issues

The *Research policy agenda for science and technology to support global health development* (1998) identified in some detail a number of important methodological issues that had been rarely or insufficiently addressed. These included use of the Internet for identifying information and collaborating on research, methods for intersectoral and behavioural research, knowledge-based health assessments, the interpretation of health data, modelling and simulation, and priority-setting. Annex 2 contains excerpts from the Research policy agenda summarizing thinking on these issues.

---

is no barrier, in principle, to the simultaneous use of both qualitative and quantitative information in the description of the system.

"An account of explicit and implicit inputs and outputs and the status of discernible components within the system, constitutes a description of it and also represents a 'model' of the system. Furthermore, it constitutes part of a relational database, which will typically include both qualitative information (including relationships) and quantitative data and relationships; the information/data can be coupled with "degrees of belief", providing for 'inexact' reasoning about the system. More particularly, the relational data base will contain rules expressing, for instance, observed associations, 'consequences' of disturbances and interventions within the system, and other behavioural characteristics.

"In the present context, the proposition is that this 'rule-based' approach to modelling will certainly circumvent the first of the two problems met by mathematical modelling, and it seems likely that the second difficulty can also be minimized by the same approach. A relational database model of a system can be readily made much more comprehensive than a fully-quantitative mathematical model, because relevant information is easier to obtain and express and because, in principle, logical analysis can draw from the input information a more comprehensive representation than could be achieved from the use of a presumed structure."

BOX 11

Themes for global health development in the Research policy agenda (1998)

Disease conditions and health impairments

Communicable/infectious diseases
- Acute respiratory infections
- Tuberculosis
- Vaccine-preventable diseases of childhood
- Diarrhoeal diseases
- Sexually transmitted diseases and AIDS
- Tropical diseases, including parasitic diseases

Non-communicable diseases
- Cancer
- Cardiovascular disease
- Diabetes
- Haemoglobin disorders, such as sickle cell disease and thalassaemia
- Musculoskeletal disorders (such as osteoarthritis, rheumatoid arthritis, osteoporosis)
- Other health impairments and conditions deserving research attention (include blindness, hearing impairment, accidents, burns and injuries, and oral health problems)
- Disabilities and impairments due to diseases and constitutional conditions, disasters, war, violence, traffic accidents, accidents in the home, occupational hazards, and excessive risk-taking behaviour
- Diagnostic, therapeutic and rehabilitative technology is needed to support programmes dealing with the entire range of communicable and "constitutional" diseases and impairments

Health systems and policies
- Primary health care
- Equitable coverage
- Health manpower and human resources
- Health policy and systems development
- International comparative research
- Quality assurance and monitoring systems
- Economic and other intersectoral policies

Family, perinatal and reproductive health
- Maternal and child health
- Perinatal health
- Child health and development
- Occupational health and safety
- Women's health and development
- Health of the elderly
- Reproductive health and family planning research

Environment and health
- "Driving forces and pressures"
- Urbanization
- Safe water supply and sanitation
- Environmental hazard monitoring and control

> ***Food and nutrition***
> - Malnutrition
> - Food production and security
> - Nutritional deficiencies
> - Micronutrient deficiencies
> - Excess nutrition or unhealthy food intake
> - Food safety
>
> ***Mental health and healthy behaviour***
> - Schizophrenic syndromes
> - Acute psychoses
> - Depressive disorders
> - Neurological disorders
> - Child mental disorders
> - Dementias
> - Substance abuse
> - Healthy behaviour
> - Suicides and parasuicides

5.4 Substantive themes

All problems of public health importance are relevant to WHO's work, particularly at global and regional levels. Research is essential to advance understanding of, and appropriate solutions, to such problems, as well as overall competency within the organization. The *Research policy agenda for science and technology to support global health development* proposed by the ACHR (1998) discussed extensively the substantive themes for global health development and advised on their relevance to WHO. A summary structure of those themes is given in Box 11.

5.5 Initiatives in formulating research strategy, 1950 2000

In terms of strategic thinking, several initiatives have featured in the life of WHO. As mentioned earlier, the late 1950s saw the birth of the ACMR and the 1960s saw the attempted creation of a World Health Research Centre.

In 1975, the ACMR held a roundtable discussion chaired by Lord S. Zuckerman, who was then a member of the committee.

Between 1983 and 1988, Prof. T. McKeown chaired a subcommittee on health research strategy which issued its formal report in 1986. However, between 1986 and 1988, the work was further refined in light of available evidence and relevant feedback. Just a few weeks before he died in June 1988, Prof. McKeown tabled an update for the following (October) session of the ACHR which is reported below.

"Research for health" was the subject of the "technical discussions" at the World Health Assembly in 1990, and a further attempt at strategy formulation took place, part of which is excerpted.

A strategy update was published in 1993 by the ACHR under the chairmanship of Prof. M. Gabr. Abstracts from this are reproduced, together with highlights from a subsequent report published in 1998 under Prof. Fliedner's chairmanship.

Also in the area of strategic thinking, the impact of scientific advances on future health was the subject of a joint colloquium, held under the aegis of the ACHR and the Council for International Organizations of Medical Sciences (CIOMS). This was attended by distinguished participants, including two Nobel laureates.

5.5.1 The Zuckerman roundtable (1975)

The concern with the formulation of a strategic approach to research was articulated in 1975 with an important ACMR roundtable meeting chaired by Lord Zuckerman, then a member of the committee.

In introducing the topic, Lord Zuckerman emphasized the importance of prioritizing health needs both in terms of their social significance and according to the possibilities of tackling them with the knowledge currently available and within the constraints set by the limitations of resources. Only once this has been done can one see what is missing.

"We are not dealing with a static situation anywhere, but a dynamic one," Lord Zuckerman said. "Time is not on our side. Population is growing. Poverty is growing. Urbanization is bringing about new environmental problems." It is becoming increasingly difficult, he added, to transfer knowledge which would help achieve WHO's objectives.

Lord Zuckerman stressed that ultimately any programme of biomedical research which becomes the policy of a country is that country's own national responsibility. Although ACMR members had agreed that biomedical research should be carried out in developing countries, he pointed out that the expertise to do this research was frequently not available. "We would be deluding ourselves if we supposed that the more sophisticated kinds of health care which the advanced countries enjoy can be immediately and easily transported to some countries of the Third World," Lord Zuckerman added.

Lord Zuckerman's statement to the 1975 roundtable meeting is reproduced in Annex 3.

In the following year (1976), WHO's governing bodies were involved in discussing WHO's role in health research. At the subsequent session of the ACMR in June 1976, a discussion on the "long-term perspectives of WHO's research programme" took place, and the committee came to certain significant conclusions.

Since the formal organization of research at WHO in 1958, there had been repeated references in the World Health Assembly (in resolution WHA28.70, for instance), and in the WHO Manual and other WHO documents, to the organization's programme of research. Resolution WHA29.64 confirmed "the need for the drawing-up of a comprehensive long-term programme for the development and coordination of biomedical and health services research" and invited "the Director-General to prepare a comprehensive report containing an analysis and evaluation of WHO's research-coordinating activities".

WHO's research activities have been planned and carried out, with few exceptions, as integral parts of the organization's programmes and not as part of an organization-wide programme of research coordinated and funded through an identifiable framework and plan.

In 1975 it was estimated that about US$ 5 million, representing less that 4% of WHO's regular budget, were allocated each year to research activities. Additional extrabudgetary funds estimated at US$ 15 million comprised the remainder of WHO's annual expenditures for research. These modest resources, through their association with WHO programmes, were considered to have a catalytic effect which substantially increased their impact.

5.5.2 *Conclusions of the McKeown Report (1988)*

The ACMR's Subcommittee on Health Research Strategy, which was chaired by Prof. T. McKeown, reported to the committee in 1985. The report was published the following year. Two years later, shortly before his death, Prof. McKeown prepared an update of the report.

The update pointed out that there were at that time "no well-recognized priorities" in the research programmes of developing countries. The failure to establish priorities, it said, was also noted in health service policies that lacked direction for research. Yet the need for priorities was clear in 1988, as illustrated in the areas of nutrition and sanitation.

Since the global population was expected to double before stabilizing, and since the population of Africa was expected to increase about six times, "on the basis of present policies it seems inevitable that serious food deficiencies will continue well into the next century," Dr McKeown stated. Similarly, he said, WHO data on sanitary progress showed that in 1988 "we are not in sight of the time when clean water and adequate sanitation will be generally available in developing countries, particularly in rural areas".

Prof McKeown compared the experience of developed countries and developing countries that have made rapid progress. In developed countries, for instance, the fall in deaths from infectious diseases resulted from increased resistance (which in turn resulted from improved nutrition and immunization) and from reduced exposure to infection. Other contributing influences were the control of fertility, improvements in education, and economic growth.

Developing countries which at the time had advanced rapidly in health were also seen to have substantially improved the nutrition of their population (though Prof. McKeown concluded that immunization had contributed "relatively little" to resistance to infection and improvements in water supply and sanitation were of limited significance in reducing exposure to infection).

"The direct influences which lead to the rapid decline of infections are (a) increase of resistance from better nutrition and immunization, and (b) reduced exposure mainly through hygienic measures," Prof. McKeown stated. Though, while all these influences had contributed to health improvements in developed countries, "to this point in time the predominant influence in the Third World was improved nutrition".

Prof. McKeown's update stressed the important role of nutrition in health but pointed out that the causes of food insecurity and the ill-health it causes are determined largely by national policies. He argued that the chief requirements were to promote food domestic production (by shifting resources from industry to agriculture, from large to small farms, from capital-intensive to labour-intensive activities) and to give people at risk of food insecurity the opportunity to earn an adequate income.

The full text of Prof. McKeown's 1988 update to the report of the ACMR Subcommittee on Health Research Strategy is reproduced in Annex 4.

5.5.3 The importance of research career structures (technical discussions at the World Health Assembly, 1990)

Of the many critical issues discussed at the 1990 technical discussions (5), and one which still receives insufficient attention, is the importance of research career structures. The discussions revealed "considerable variability" between countries' capacities to use the results of health research, and concluded that one important key to successful research – and adoption of research findings – was a clear career structure for researchers.

The recommendations that emerged referred to the need for good candidates to be attracted to a research career, for reasonable pay and benefits for researchers, and for a system of promotion and career progression. This could be achieved, it was proposed, by setting up a "civil-service type structure" for research workers, by treating them as general public service staff but with a research subsidy, or by putting them on a career scale similar to that of university teachers.

The recommendations of the technical discussions on research career structures are reproduced in Annex 5.

5.5.4 New methodologies and the need to better understand the economic environment

The publication *Research for health: principles, perspectives and strategies* (18) was a concise but comprehensive report which, for the first time, emphasized the need for new methodologies and for a better understanding of the economic environment. The report argued that the WHO definition of health recognizes that it is a complex concept and cannot be regarded simply as the absence of overt disease or disability. Other aspects that must be taken into account include quality of life, protection against biological and psychosocial health-damaging assaults, the intensity and nature of risks to health, the presence of health defects and health-relevant deficits.

Hitherto, only limited attention had been given – when identifying sources of harm to health or the means to promote health – to determining priorities for research or formulating health research strategy. Economic and psychosocial influences on health, for instance, needed clearer elucidation, while understanding behavioural factors – both health-promoting and health-damaging – could provide an important basis for influencing community health.

Annex 6 provides an extract from *Research for health: principles, perspectives and strategies* which reveals the full scope of the document.

5.5.5 The impact of scientific advances on future health (1994)

The colloquium on "The impact of scientific advances on future health" was convened in 1994 with the aim of identifying and documenting the most critical, current and potential developments in science that were likely to have a major impact on medicine and public health over the next 20 years.

The introductory key papers presented an interpretation of the state of science at the time with respect to public health and human development. The discussion of basic science centred on DNA technologies since it was recognized that these technologies – and molecular biology in general – represented the most important and significant advances in the sciences relative to health. Such technologies were beginning to be applied to the investigation, treatment and control of many major health problems.

The colloquium felt that products generated by biotechnology were too expensive and that affordable products were needed. Participants felt that emerging controls on research threatened to restrict the growth of research, but it was stressed that any application of DNA technologies to humans should be conducted with respect to privacy and ethical conduct. Efforts to explore and expand applications in diagnosis, therapy, prevention and investigation of pathogenesis of diseases were encouraged. It was stated that the ethical aspects of somatic gene therapy had raised no new issues, but that germ line therapy should be discouraged. WHO and CIOMS, together with other international organizations, were recommended to continue working towards an international agreement on a code of ethics in molecular biology – especially on the human genome project (see *Further reading*).

The recommendations from the colloquium on "The impact of scientific advances on future health" are included in Annex 7.

5.5.6 Research policy agenda for science and technology to support global health development (1998)

The *Research policy agenda* took a forward-looking view of health research in a context of global cooperation between the scientific community, governments, NGOs and other partners in public health. At the core of the agenda were six points, namely:

1. In spite of diversity, there is a common fate, condition and ethic of all humanity that unifies action for global health development.
2. While most health impacts are "local", many underlying causes and potential solutions are "global" and multifactorial in nature.
3. Global health challenges, problems and determinants call for a more systematic global approach in support of action at international, national and local levels.
4. The world's scientists and scientific institutions must work together and with all relevant partners, not only in conventional "biomedical research", but in all research that contributes to health.
5. "Intelligent" research networks need to be expanded or developed around major issues, taking advantage of appropriate communications technologies.
6. A continuous process for definition, planning, implementation and evaluation of global research imperatives and opportunities is required.

A detailed summary of the future of health research as envisioned in the *Research policy agenda* is contained in Annex 8.

6. Regional contributions to health-related research

Regional involvement in health research constitutes a critical development in WHO's efforts to promote and coordinate research.

There are several reasons why these initiatives were important, most notably because of the following:

- The establishment of administrative focal points within the regional offices identified research promotion and development as a priority area and created the need for special expertise in research management.
- Each regional office became equipped with a formal top-level scientific advisory structure (the Advisory Committee on Medical Research, to be renamed ACHR in 1986), which had cross-representations with the global committee (the global chair attending regional meetings and vice-versa).
- Cooperation with medical research councils (MRCs) and analogous bodies became a necessity since they were usually the national decision-making bodies for setting priorities and funding. Joint meetings between regional ACHRs and MRCs were often held, thus drawing more attention to the science and technology establishment.
- The regionalization of research promoted more contacts with universities and academia, whereas the traditional communication of WHO had been mainly with Ministries of Health. It became necessary as well to involve country offices in research matters.
- Research capacity strengthening became an overarching objective. Several initiatives derived from this, for example, expanded efforts in research training, in supporting national research projects, in promoting health systems research and essential national research and in advocating the need for research career structures.

The following sections are summary accounts of principal developments in the WHO regions and do not attempt to portray specifically the precise course of events. These accounts (below) cover periods extending beyond the main scope of this history. They are presented in order to make the regional evolutions intelligible, given their relatively recent (with the exception of PAHO) involvement in research. More detailed reports can be found elsewhere (e.g. on the web sites of the WHO regional offices).

6.1 WHO AFRICAN REGION

6.1.1 Introduction

Post-independence Africa was plagued with many health problems: infectious, parasitic, nutritional and environmental catastrophes. Very high maternal and childhood morbidity coupled with rapidly occurring pregnancies often led to recurrent abortions and stillbirths, while up to the 1960s there were no efficient tools for prevention, diagnosis, treatment or control of most of the illnesses. Severe foci of river blindness and sleeping sickness led to important migrations. There were frequent and severe outbreaks of smallpox, measles and meningitis, whereas the tools to deal with these events – health infrastructure, trained health personnel, equipment, supplies and even the general organization and distribution of health services – were all grossly insufficient. The little research that was done was carried out almost exclusively by expatriates as there was hardly any indigenous research capacity. In the light of such a situation, action by WHO on multiple fronts was of urgent necessity.

The African Advisory Committee on Medical/Health Research (AACHR) was established in 1976 with a view to strengthening research capacity in the African Region. However, research funds and facilities were critically lacking at national levels while African regional budget was insufficient to remedy this situation. Bilateral agencies often followed their own research agendas that did not always take into account the countries' needs and priorities. It is therefore not surprising that the AACHR welcomed the creation of special programmes and their extrabudgetary funding to cover the needs of the region.

6.1.2 Special research programmes

Following the creation in the 1970s of HRP and TDR, WHO also created regional research components of its headquarters programmes such as those on mental health, diarrhoeal diseases control, the expanded programme on immunization, acute respiratory infections, health systems research and health manpower development. The headquarters Global Programme on AIDS was also extended to Africa and the AACHR became part of the African Advisory Committee for Health Development (AACHD).

TDR, and to a great extent HRP, with their independent technical committees became the principal agents for strengthening research capability in a large number of research institutions (institutes, councils, university faculties of science and of medicine) while, over the years, 40% of TDR's annual grants were allocated to young researchers. Assistance was provided to strengthen research institutions, many of which became centres of excellence and remain so to date. Meetings of directors of research bodies were organized while expert groups defined research priorities in fields of concern. Between 1978 and 1983, the Strengthening Health Research Services programme (SHRS) based in Abidjan, with financial support from USAID, ran a series of training workshops in English and French (first focused on research methodology, they soon expanded into protocol development). Training of health personnel in research activities and data collection received special attention; promising young researchers were identified for further training.

The take-off of HSR remained rather slow, with problems specific to each country, while the degree of priority varies greatly. As of 1990 a new concept appeared – essential National Health Research (ENHR) – leading to the creation of the Council of Health Research for Development (COHRED) which continues to work with many African countries, particularly to define goals and plans for strengthening national research capacities.

6.1.3 Health research

As of the 1980s "health for all" became the overall goal of WHO activities. The AACHR developed its own research strategy (the "scenario") within the regional initiative known as the African Health Development Framework. It focused on finding alternative solutions for the implementation of primary health care. The triad of research, management and training at the three levels of the health system formed a major part of the programme. The organization of research focal points within national ministries of health was hampered by budgetary restrictions at national and regional levels, and activities were financed mainly by extrabudgetary funds (e.g. the Netherlands supported programmes in 14 countries).

Health research in Africa thus evolved over the years as the different programmes were implemented, relying heavily on the contribution of TDR. Training, building research teams, partnerships, linkages, infrastructure development and improved communication were all supported by TDR in order to enhance the capacity of the countries to carry out research in the target diseases. Long-term (five years) grants were awarded on a sliding scale to institutions with acceptable programmes during which the trained scientists would initiate the research. Young scientists would be suitably identified, recruited and sent for training, often at PhD level. On their return they would resume their positions in the institution, enhancing local research capacities. Thus, a critical mass of researchers was slowly built up in the countries. With the increasing complexity and competition for the limited funds available, TDR developed a flexible approach to meet the special needs of the least developed countries that had previously been underserved. This strategy was successful and led to the rapid and successful development of a number of research institutions headed by well-trained nationals.

6.1.4 AACHR support to specific programmes

In the process of developing the research component of several national or international health programmes, the AACHR was a resource organization for a lot of institutions doing research on malaria, schistosomiasis, leishmaniasis, HIV/AIDS and other diseases. Other institutions received substantial research support from TDR.

The Multilateral Initiative on Malaria in Africa (MIM) is a research programme that contributed positively to furthering good research and capacity development in many African countries. It was established in 1997 by TDR in collaboration with other partners, with the overarching goal of strengthening and sustaining, through collaborative research and training, the capability of malaria endemic countries to carry out the research required to develop or improve tools for malaria control. Following the Alma-Ata

Declaration on Health For All in 1978, the emphasis was put on the development of basic health services, and health research was recognized as a necessary and critical tool in the reorganization of national health services based on primary health care. The WHO Regional Office for Africa supported these efforts with bilateral partners such as USAID and, later on, the Netherlands. This resulted in a programme based in Harare, Zimbabwe, involving five East and Southern African countries (and later the whole region) through local workshops with a strong emphasis on learning by doing. In spite of real progress in research capacity-building, the extent and nature of competence in health systems research varied with the countries' levels of socioeconomic development.

6.1.5 Sustainability versus brain-drain: a great challenge for Africa

Scientists returning to their home institutions after long studies abroad usually require support and encouragement to put into practice their newly acquired knowledge and to train younger researchers. TDR made a special provision for re-entry grants in order to avoid a brain-drain of researchers wishing to remain abroad rather than return home. TDR training grants always focused on each trainee having a staff position in his/her institution to which he/she would return after training, plus an ongoing research agenda and support in the institution into which the trainees would fit on return.

6.1.6 Conclusion

The last three decades bear witness to the considerable advances in training researchers and developing institutional capacity in African countries, and especially the least developed countries. The WHO Regional Office for Africa and other agencies have been involved in this effort. Institutions and researchers are now more responsive to the needs of their countries with regard to training in research. A new generation has emerged to direct disease control at national level. Many of them work with research partners in industrialized countries on an equal footing and play leading roles in strengthening research capacity in other countries in their region. Multidisciplinary teams continue to be built up and some of the strengthened institutions are located in rural areas where the disease burden is greatest. However, much remains to be done: health systems and policy research, as well as the problem of the interface between research results and health policy and implementation, still has to be dealt with adequately. The dialogue between researchers and policy-makers seems to have started and policy-makers are beginning to commission research.

The major drawback remains the persistent dependence of African Member States on external funding. The health research under the auspices of the WHO Regional Office for Africa is also enhanced through interregional activities. The Alliance for Health Policy and Systems Research, an initiative of the Global Forum for Health Research (GFHR) works in close collaboration with WHO. It focuses its efforts on strengthening health policy as well as health systems research with a strong thrust on enhancing health system performance in developing countries. GFHR is a Swiss-based foundation with an international vision. It was created in 1996 following the report of an ad hoc committee set up after the publication of the World Bank *World development report*

1993 which emphasized the role of research in development. GFHR has thus been promoting research globally with emphasis on stimulating research on health problems affecting poorer communities.

6.2 WHO EASTERN MEDITERRANEAN REGION

WHO's Regional Office for the Eastern Mediterranean has been involved in assisting and promoting medical and health research since 1966. However, with the establishment in 1976 of a regional programme for research promotion and development, these collaborative activities were intensified. Political commitment started growing, national coordinating mechanisms were established and allocations were made for research in WHO collaborative programmes. Nevertheless, it was felt that intensified efforts were needed to enable Member States to develop their health research systems further and to use research increasingly to provide evidence for policy-making and health actions, especially in reducing health inequalities and in addressing the health problems of the poorer segments of the population.

6.2.1 *The Eastern Mediterranean Advisory Committee for Health Research*

The Regional Office for the Eastern Mediterranean has been involved in medical research since the first informal meeting held in Alexandria in 1966. This meeting strongly recommended a programme of research relevant to specific needs of the countries with a plan of work for further promotion of health research within the region. For this purpose an Eastern Mediterranean Advisory Committee on Biomedical Research (EMACBR) was formed in 1976 and became in 1982 the Eastern Mediterranean Committee on Health Research (EMACHR). This comprises a balanced (in terms of both geography and expertise) group of senior and outstanding researchers from the region. They serve in their individual capacities for a term of three to four years (sometimes extendable). The committee has the mandate to provide advice to the Regional Director (as deemed necessary by him) on all matters related to health research and development in the region. It performs its consultative mandate in accordance with the terms of reference given by the Regional Director. So far, 23 sessions of the EMACHR have been held since its inception and quite intensive activities have been undertaken by the regional office covering almost every aspect of the research needs of the region. The emerging recommendations of the committee advised leadership on how to ensure an appropriate scientific and technical input to the evolving programmes in the region and on the mechanisms that could be used to promote and put into operation the necessary research activities.

6.2.2 *Research Policy and Cooperation unit*

A Research Promotion and Development (RPD) unit was established by the WHO Regional Office for the Eastern Mediterranean in 1978, was renamed as the Research Policy and Strategy Coordination (RPS) unit in 1998, and subsequently became the Research Policy and Cooperation (RPC) unit. This unit maintains close contacts with its counterparts at WHO headquarters and in other regions, as well as with national focal points for research, medical research councils and major health research institutions in the Eastern Mediterranean Region. The RPC unit works in close collaboration with other technical units of the regional office and other national and international partners. The unit also serves as the secretariat for the EMACHR. Over the years, the RPC unit has promoted research and capacity-building – especially health systems research – through national and regional training programmes.

6.2.3 Promotion of effective health systems in Member States

Through site visits, the health research potential of several Member States was assessed and areas of collaboration determined. A system for the award of grants for research and research training was set up. Research priorities in different programmes were identified. To promote collaborative research activities a large number of institutions were designated as WHO collaborating centres. An active programme was initiated for training in research methodology, research management and scientific writing. The coordination of research in the region was facilitated through meetings of representatives of research councils or of analogous bodies and through close contacts with WHO's global programmes for research and research training.

The establishment of the *Eastern Mediterranean health journal* in 1986 facilitated the publication of results of research by scientists in the region. A task force visited 10 countries between 1986 and 1994 to promote and develop national plans for research in support of national strategies for health for all by the year 2000.

Meanwhile, the regional office has been actively involved in funding research proposals received from within the region as well as in assisting Member States to strengthen their capacity and set their priorities to undertake health research with a view to improving their health research systems. The overall research support and capacity-building efforts of the regional office over the last few decades were:

— research for health funding;
— training manpower;
— building research infrastructure;
— linking research to local health priorities;
— health research strategies and policies.

Research for health funding

The EMACHR at its 1977 session strongly recommended the establishment of a "special biomedical research fund" and proposed the development of a regional programme for submission to governments for financing on a voluntary basis. However, until 1992, the proposals were supported by the regional office on an ad hoc basis and dealt with a wide range of topics. A small grants scheme was established in 1992 in collaboration with TDR. A similar scheme was planned with the HRP programme.

A unit on Research in the Communicable Diseases was established in 1992 in order to support researchers from the Eastern Mediterranean Region in addressing local problems in disease control, as well as to raise the research capacity of regional researchers in operational research with implication for the control programme. The scheme was primarily funded by Arab funds and was later supported by the WHO Regional Office for the Eastern Mediterranean, UNDP/World Bank/WHO, TDR, the WHO Division of Control of Tropical Diseases (CTD), and Roll Back Malaria (RBM). Research was initially limited to topics of regional specificity (e.g. malaria, schistosomiasis, tuberculosis, leishmaniasis and lymphatic filariasis). In 2002 the scope of the scheme expanded to include other communicable diseases such as HIV, sexually transmitted diseases, vaccine preventable diseases, haemorrhagic fevers, brucellosis, meningitis and echinococcosus. Thus, with a modest budget, the scheme provided an opportunity for researchers to address local problems that might not receive attention at the global level. More than 340 proposals have been funded under this scheme since 1992.

In 2002 a new grant for research in priority areas of public health was established by the regional office, with the aim of addressing local problems and issues of public health importance with special emphasis on health systems research. Through a competitive process of selection, funds of up to US$ 10,000 were provided to successful research proposals. The duration of research under this grant is generally around one year. Some 140 research proposals have been supported in Eastern Mediterranean Member States in six rounds of research funded under this programme.

The regional office, in partnership with the Standing Committee for Science and Technology of the Organization of Islamic Countries (COMSTECH), established in 2004 a special grant for research in applied biotechnology and genomics. The overall aim of the grant was to promote research, encourage networking, generate new knowledge and stimulate the application of biotechnology and genomic-driven interventions in health care. The priority areas for research were chosen and 35 proposals from the Member States were supported in two rounds of research funded by the regional office and COMSTECH.

Training manpower

Human resource development in health research is among the key strategies emphasized in the "Renewed Policy for Health Research and Development in the Region". The regional office supports training in health research at both national and regional levels. In 1977 a committee was formed to support training and research activities in the fields of health systems research. After 1990, the regional programme for Research Promotion and Development focused more on the development of multidisciplinary manpower and institutional bases for research, with promotion of research management and coordination at the national level, and intercountry collaboration in areas of common concern. For capacity-building in health research in the region, several international, regional and national training workshops were organized that addressed such topics as grant proposal writing, research policy and practice, health research priority setting, situation analysis of health research, health research ethical review process, exploring demand for health research by national policy-makers and writing research articles for publication.

In recent years, the regional office has further enhanced its efforts for capacity-building in research for health, especially in research methodology, clinical research, writing of research proposals and scientific papers, community-based research for health and user-driven research. So far more than 500 health researchers from almost all countries of the region have been trained.

Building research infrastructure

The situation analysis of health research in the region highlights the insufficient development of integrated, well designed and functioning national health research systems. However, from the information collected it appears that a well developed infrastructure for health research exists in most countries and some useful research is being carried out both in specialized centres and in academic situations. Nevertheless, there is a dire need to strengthen the existing systems to improve the quantity and quality of demand-oriented research for health and to develop mechanisms to translate research results into policy.

For quick reference of health researchers, scholars, policy-makers and other stakeholders of health services, a database on regional institutional capacity in genomics and biotechnology was made available by the regional office on the Internet in 2005. Further development of the database on institutional capacity for conducting research in the region is continued by extending the information to several other aspects of health research.

Linking research to local health priorities

To overcome the lack of health research systems in the region, linking research to local health priorities has always been one of the priority areas for the "special grant for research in priority areas of public health" since 2002. Unfortunately, despite these efforts, the situation of the health services and systems research has shown a negligible improvement in quantity and quality. Recently the regional office enhanced its activities for strengthening national priority-setting for health research and, in this regard, the researchers and policy-makers in at least five countries of the region will be trained in methods of priority-setting.

Health research strategies and policies

In spite of constant efforts throughout the years, it was recognized at the turn of the century that research activities and programmes are still fragmented with a lot of duplication and a lack of focus on national needs and priorities. This led to the emergence of a vision of a systems approach to health research driven by equity, focused on national goals and priorities, and operating within an interactive regional and global framework. This prospect was supported by the Ministerial Summit on Health Research convened by WHO and held in Mexico City in 2004. The summit statement called for the generation of knowledge to improve health through strengthening health systems, utilization of research results for policy and action, and for attainment of national and global Millennium Development Goals. It also emphasized better communication, information-sharing and knowledge dissemination as a means of improving national health research capacity, especially in developing countries. Following this global conference, WHO Regional Office for the Eastern Mediterranean organized several meetings (e.g. regional consultations, expert groups, ministerial fora) in order to enhance countries' research capacities, to bridge the gap between scientific knowledge and operationalization of research results to improve the health of the people, and to develop a research culture in ministries of health.

6.2.4 Research ethics

The critical role of ethical guidelines in health care and research is not only well recognized as essential for ensuring equity but also for protecting individuals and communities from unnecessary risks and harm. Given the regional social, cultural and religious norms, each region must have its own set of guidelines and regulations which Member States can draw upon to define codes of ethical practice. This has been stated explicitly by the WHO Regional Office for the Eastern Mediterranean on several occasions and at policy level by the EMACBR.

Many countries have developed a core ethical framework for health care and research ethics. The overall direction of this development has been within the context of religious, social and cultural practices in the region, while at the same time embracing other nations' ethical values and principles that are not in conflict with the local value systems. The Islamic Organization for Medical Sciences (IOMS) and the Gulf Cooperation Council (GCC) are the two leading entities currently at the forefront of advocacy, increasing awareness for the need to develop ethical review mechanisms. Several countries have already developed capacities in health ethics, with properly instituted review and regulation processes. They have created national ethical review committees, most of which follow WHO published guidelines on ethics in health care and research, though other guidelines such as the Helsinki Declaration and the Nuremberg Code are also being used by some ethical review committees. Publication of relevant documents and the organization of training activities have been complemented by a Masters degree in bioethics initiated by the regional office in partnership with the University of Toronto, Canada.

6.2.5 Web site of the Research Policy and Cooperation unit of the regional office

The RPC unit launched its web site in 2005 to reflect the efforts carried out by the regional office and to encourage wider involvement of Member States in applied health research, through promoting health systems research, supporting research grants, capacity-building and consultations in health research. The site also highlights the health research policies, programmes and other activities of the regional office. It provides links to some useful related websites and serves as a source of instant information for research funding and training opportunities both from within WHO and from other sources.

6.2.6 Conclusion

The overall weak state of health research in the region and its limited ability to influence national policies call for a thorough revision of existing research strategies of WHO at global and regional levels. Any such strategy must be based on rigorous methods to assess evidence to guide the decision-making process: do new interventions offer cost-effective improvements for public health?

As considerable effort and time would be needed to make sure the best evidence can be applied in practice, special research would be needed on how to shorten this time and optimize the resources needed for this purpose. Consequently, the regional office will continue capacity-building and support for research for health in the Member States. This support will be aimed at:

— providing health research policy support and advice to Member States;
— further strengthening countries' health research capacities by supplying research grants in health systems research and in applied biotechnology;
— offering training facilities to improve the quality of research for health, addressing priorities and improving capacities in research ethics;
— building capacities and mechanisms for effective utilization of research results;
— undertaking situation analysis of health research systems in several countries of the region;
— engaging stakeholders in regional research efforts;
— developing further collaboration and partnerships with international health research organizations, universities and other partners.

Notwithstanding this ambitious programme, it is obvious that even the best evidence will only help if translated into real policies by governance bodies.

6.3 WHO EUROPEAN REGION

6.3.1 Introduction

The WHO European Region is made up of 57 countries. A major change in the region resulted from the fall of the Berlin wall in 1989. Europe has a long tradition of medical research with great differences between countries. Like other WHO regions, Europe has been dramatically affected by the HIV/AIDS epidemic. The Chernobyl catastrophe was a European modern plague whose ill-effects are still underestimated. Another specificity is the existence of the European Union: many European countries are members of this political grouping that includes a wide range of research on many problems concerned with the health and well-being of Europeans. These unique characteristics play an important role in the work and prerogatives of the WHO Regional Office for Europe and are reflected in the history of medical and health research.

6.3.2 Analytical review

Created in 1976, the European Advisory Committee on Medical Research (EACMR, and now EACHR) has been active in three dimensions: within WHO as a whole it promotes coordination and exchanges on research with the global and other regional research committees; within the WHO Regional Office for Europe it stimulates research in the various sectors and departments; and in Europe it collects, exchanges and uses information in the region. Taking into account that classical medical research was reasonably well established in European countries in the 1970s, the EACMR concentrated on methods of promoting health services research. Because of the different systems of health care in the various countries, there were obvious difficulties in internationalizing that type of research, whereas other types of biomedical research more readily transcended national boundaries. With a view to overcoming these obstacles five subgroups were established, namely: standardization of techniques for identifying a defined population; preventive measures and critical review of the routine check-ups; designing output indicators; health economics (is the cost-benefit approach reliable?) and evaluation of new drugs. In 1978, after a consultation of Member States and European medical research councils, hypertension (as related to health care delivery) was selected as one of the topics for coordinated research. Member States were requested to express the nature and extent of possible support and cooperation.

Two years after its start, the EACMR was already operational, having defined its priority areas and way of proceeding, and having found its niche in European medical research. The first liaison meeting on health research coordination within the WHO European Region took place in September 1979. UNESCO, the Commission of European Communities and several national research institutions participated.

The 1978 WHO-UNICEF conference in Alma-Ata was important as the concept of primary health care, proposed by WHO, was universally endorsed with the ambitious objective of "health for all by the year 2000" (HFA 2000). Following the Alma-Ata declaration, the WHO Regional Office for Europe prepared a programme with 38 targets for the implementation of HFA 2000 and the committee reviewed it extensively with the mandate to advise the regional office. Three working groups were formed to review the sections on lifestyles conducive to health, a healthy environment, and appropriate care. These groups gave comments on how to improve the document and outlined problem areas requiring further scientific work. They proposed the contents for a research chapter, and these were expanded in 1984. The committee dealt extensively with the research needs of a health-for-all strategy. It was once more recognized that unhealthy lifestyles and environmental pollution may well impair health. In 1978, the word "medical" in the title of the committee was replaced by "health". The EACHR stressed the necessity to distinguish short-, medium- and long-term goals regarding the improvement of existing knowledge and development of new knowledge.

The EACHR involvement in the development of a research policy for HFA 2000 increased with the adoption of the 38 regional targets by the WHO Regional Committee for Europe in 1984. The EACHR analysed the research implications of the regional strategy target by target and a revised version of the research plan was presented to the Regional Committee in 1986. The same year, after the Chernobyl accident, a regional office programme was developed for one epidemiological survey, including follow-up of the early and long-term effects of accidental radiation releases and the accumulation of radioactive nuclides in the environment and food, as well as for public health awareness and early warning for accidents. The EACHR urged increased priority for environmental health research and gave high priority to risk assessment and management. In 1988 a special programme on AIDS focused on the development of an epidemiological surveillance system in cooperation with the Commission of European Communities (CEC).

The cooperation with other organizations was intensified. Reports were received from the European medical research councils and the Health Research Committee of the European Community. Both were prepared to use the regional research plan for health for all as a source of inspiration.

The early 1990s saw consolidation following the major economic and social changes taking place in Europe, particularly in the countries of Central and Eastern Europe (CCEE). These new developments also changed the order of priorities for regional health policies and for health research policies as well. Consequently the main objective of the EACHR became how to support the development of health research policies and strengthen health research capacities for the CCEE countries. The following years were a difficult period for the EACHR, which was working in economically stringent conditions due to the region wide recession. The dramatic changes made the issues of health research a less important priority and more attention was needed to generate the response to large-scale acute health problems in CCEE and in the Newly Independent States (NIS). Notwithstanding, the regional office's Division of Environmental Health carried out an extensive study among all European countries on several aspects of environment and health, resources, institutions, policy and research priorities. The results were published by the regional office in 1994 in *Concern for Europe's tomorrow*. These data had a strong impact on the Environment and Health Action Plan for Europe (EHAP) that was discussed in 1994 by the 47 European ministers of environment and health who adopted a Declaration on Environment and Health. During the same period, a Research Policy Agenda was prepared under the direction of Professor Fliedner, chairman of the EACHR. Published in 1997,this has inspired many research programmes within and outside WHO.

6.3.3 A new era

In 1997, the EACHR's first priority became the provision of scientific input and the evidence base for preparation of the renewed health-for-all strategy. The 1998 meeting went deeper into the concept of the evidence base, inaugurating a long process of work on this new approach to health problems. This was not the first time that the WHO European Region became interested in evidence: in the 1980s, the preparation of the European health-for-all plan was strongly evidence-based, and the EACHR contributed directly to this development. The WHO roles envisaged within this plan implied that work on the evidence base would need to be ongoing. The emphasis was put on increasing health knowledge and the production and use of meaningful information. However, the concept of evidence, initially coming from clinical medicine, was to be scientifically reinforced and applied to the field of public health. The EACHR meeting in 1998 underlined the unevenness in the existence of evidence, noting in particular the relative scarcity of evidence on the effectiveness of community-based public health action and on the implementation of policy into practice. It stated that the current evidence base was by no means exhaustive but was rather a first step. This implies that the search for and analysis of international evidence should proceed in using a common nomenclature, having dedicated staff, and combined with its review and rating by public health specialists, networks and programme managers, in order to allow continuous adjustment of international health action and WHO statements in light of the evidence. The EACHR worked as an observer and a promoter of evidence for health development. The 1998 meeting appears as a turning point between on one hand the former committee of which it was the last session and, on the other, the first gathering of the renewed EACHR in 2001. Fortunately enough, even in the absence of formal meetings in-between, there was a progressive maturation of the concept of evidence base.

Meanwhile a lot of transformations took place in Europe and plenty of initiatives in the regional office helped to adapt it to the new geopolitical situation. Fruitful external contacts were developed with WHO headquarters, Member States, consultants and members of the scientific community, allowing the momentum in theoretical progress and practical applications to be maintained. The emphasis on the evidence basis was reinforced as an important means for meeting the challenge of health-for-all in a new and complex situation.

For the renewed EACHR, the period 2001–2007 was a very busy and productive one. It began with the discussion on a draft paper on evidence for public health. The challenge was met through the publication in the *International Journal of Technology Assessment in Health Care* of a comprehensive and well-structured article titled "Considerations in defining evidence for public health" (H. David Banta, 19/3, 2003, 559-572, 52 references). This work, published under the auspices of the EACHR with the 11 members of the committee, constituted a clear and almost exhaustive statement of the state of the art at that time. The paper stated that "the issue of evidence in public health is quite complex. No existing model is adequate to the task of answering all the important questions concerning evidence and public health. Enough is known, however, to make considerable progress while working for methodological developments." This clarification proved to be helpful, and its impact widely exceeded the limits of the regional office: in fact, it was the starting point of a further deepening of the notion and use of evidence in public health. It was an extremely useful resource in itself, for it explored useful ideas about the nature of evidence, including the place of experience and anecdote. "Evidence has to be contextualized," stated the EACHR article, and this point was discussed in depth. It is obvious that, for various reasons, some countries are open-minded towards this approach to health problems while others are not. The political, social, administrative and financial parameters; the historical background, the health status of the population of any given country and its health system are all to be taken into consideration. The Regional Director thanked the committee saying that the EACHR had been a very helpful part of an undoubtedly increasing awareness of the importance of using evidence in all divisions of regional office.

In 2005 the committee was charged with including a new discussion topic – health intelligence – in employing a process similar to the way evidence had previously been addressed. Since the process had worked so well, and there were concrete results in the evidence work, in terms of both a cultural change and building up tools and procedures, it was proposed that the committee should follow the same process for developing the newcomer. This process included a conceptual discussion on the definition of health intelligence in the context of WHO in Europe, and the implementation of this concept to improve the regional office's capacity to provide guidance; a policy paper on the concept and understanding of intelligence that could guide staff in their daily work; and a programme of work in order to encourage Member States in this process in a public health approach.

The next steps included developing a position paper that capture the practical aspects of implementing a health intelligence service within the WHO Regional Office for Europe.

Significant progress was made in 2006 through the identification of three elements which the regional office was trying to integrate: data, in the form of a health-for-all database and other integrated databases, information (notably products such as the *Highlights* on health in each Member State, the *European health report* and management of web-based information); and intelligence or "actionable information" as provided by the regional office's Health Evidence Network (HEN) and the European Observatory on Health Systems and Policies.

Two of WHO's six core functions in Europe have to do with evidence and information, and strengthening the intelligence function was the second of 11 development processes put forward by the Regional Director for his 2005–2010 programme.

In spite of obvious progress, these concepts of knowledge, evidence context, health intelligence and their operationalization still require a collective and strong commitment. In order to best contribute to this endeavour, the EACHR adopted new terms of reference in 2007. The first paragraph is quite explicit: the regional office is actively entering a new phase which has been termed "health intelligence". One of the main aims of this effort is to give Member States and public health professionals easy access to intelligence related to specific public health activities. In this context, the regional office would like to help ensure that staff and programmes use the best available evidence in providing advice on intelligence to Member States.

6.3.4 Fit for the future

Could one consider that the EACHR has carried out its role and fulfilled its commitments? It has, in two different ways. A first period, 1976–1998, was devoted to installing the committee and to the inception of its work. It had to find its place within the regional office, the staff, the various programmes and vis-à-vis the Regional Committee which represents Member States. This was quite a challenge and was met in a practical way. In meeting after meeting, the regional office addressed regional health priorities and helped partners to progress in health planning, defining priorities in health research and promoting a wise utilization of research results. It played a crucial role in the building of the health-for-all strategy.

The second period, from 2001 to today, has been distinct and somewhat original. Besides its traditional missions, the EACHR developed a conceptual approach to the definition and implementation of public health, serving as a think-tank. The confident relationships with Member States, WHO headquarters and the rich scientific potential of Europe helped the regional office to define some basic and more modern concepts and to work on their practical application at various levels – international, national and local.

6.4 WHO SOUTH-EAST ASIA REGION

6.4.1 Background

The South-East Asia Regional Advisory Committee on Medical Research (SEA/ACMR) was established in 1976. Though there had been no organized medical research in the South-East Asian countries, medical and health workers conducted research on their own. For instance, Ronald Ross in India researched malaria in the 19th century, Whitmori in Yangon discovered *Pfeiferella whitmori* in 1911, and there are many other examples. With the roots of research already present in India in 1911, the India Council of Medical Research was established in 1949. Since 1964, research councils or analogous bodies have been established in many countries in South-East Asia.

Regionalization of medical research in WHO began in the 1970s initiated and guided by Director-General Dr. Halfdan Mahler. Accordingly SEA/ACMR was set up in 1976 following Regional Committee resolutions in 1973, 1974 and 1975. The secretariat included a regional adviser (medical research), a technical officer and others. SEA/ACMR had its own budget for research which, at the peak in 1988–1989 was US$ 5.97 million (US$ 3.4 million in intercountry programmes and US$ 2.57 million in country budgets).

When the research programme was in full swing, the regional Research Promotion and Development programme/intercountry programme budget was divided between support for SEA/ACMR and its secretariat, support for research programmes, and support for research capacity strengthening.

In addition to the regional budget, research in the region received support from technical divisions of WHO headquarters – especially programmes on vector biology and control, malaria, leprosy, tuberculosis, essential drugs, communicable diseases and epidemiology training, maternal and child health and family planning, and special programmes such as TDR and HRP. Also, there were sizeable inputs to research from other sources – such as the United Nations (agencies such as UNDP, UNFPA, UNAIDS) and the US Centers for Disease Control and Prevention.

The objectives of SEA/ACMR were:

— to strengthen national research capabilities;
— to promote and coordinate research on regional priorities and problems related to socioeconomic development not adequately covered by national and other efforts;
— to promote research designed to facilitate rapid application of existing and emerging scientific knowledge.

Members of SEA/ACMR were to be invited from among research scientists and managers, and experts in medicine, health and related subjects. Each member serves for four years except the chair, whose term of office is five years. There were 11 members of SEA/ACMR in 1976, from various disciplines and from six different countries. Prof. C. Gopalan from India was the first chair of SEA/RACMR. The committee reviewed and confirmed its terms of reference, the members discussed the criteria for selection of priorities for regional research, and identified six priority areas for research. These priorities include: communicable diseases (with six priority diseases), nutrition, human fertility, environmental health, delivery of health services, and others depending upon the national priorities.

At the first session of SEA/ACMR, a number of research working groups were formed, notably on health services delivery, malaria, leprosy, dengue haemorrhagic fever and later on nutrition, diarrhoea and liver diseases.

Prof. C. Gopalan chaired SEA/ACMR from 1976 to 1980 and guided it in systematic structuring and functioning. The committee underwent a consolidation phase under the chairmanship of Prof. A. A. Loedin (1981–1983) and Prof. Prawase Wasi (1984–1987). In 1985, a special session was held to commemorate the 10th anniversary of the founding of SEA/ACMR. In 1987 SEA/ACMR was renamed SEA/ACHR. The next chairpersons were Dr. S. D. M. Fermando (1988–1991) and Dr. (Mrs) Sneh Bhagava (1992–1994). The chairmanship of Dr. Aree Valyswawi (1995–1997) saw the deterioration of the global political situation, coupled with a global economic crisis, with WHO also facing great challenges. Dr. Aree had to turn these challenges into opportunities for SEA/ACHR. In 1995 a special commemorative anniversary session of the committee was held at the regional office in New Delhi. Following brief periods of chairmanship of Dr. Brotowesis (1998) and Prof. M. P. Strestha (1999), SEA/ACMR came under Prof. N. K. Ganguly as chairperson (2000–2007).

6.4.2 *National research capability strengthening*

The regional office strengthened the research capability of countries through well known mechanisms such as the following:

a) **Grants for institutional strengthening.** Research grants, research training grants, and fellowships were provided and WHO collaborating centres were designated. Medical research councils and analogous bodies were fostered in countries and were used particularly effectively as important mechanisms to promote and support research in the region. Many of the above did not take place in isolation but in the context of broad research areas.
b) **WHO collaborating centres.** Centres of excellence already existed in countries of the region, many of which were designated WHO collaborating centres. There were 85 collaborating centres in the region in 2001 and many more are being designated.
c) **Medical research councils and analogous bodies.** The regional office strengthened national bodies whose functions were to develop national policies and strategies, and to coordinate, manage and promote health research. Medical research councils have now been established in nine of the 11 member countries of the South-East Asia Region. WHO is the only international organization in the region that has consistently strengthened medical research councils.

6.4.3 *Promotion, coordination and support of regional priority research projects*

Criteria were established by the regional office in 1976 for setting priorities in supporting health research. Approximately 253 research projects were funded by the regional office during the first and second decade of the committee but the numbers declined considerably later.

Most research projects were concerned with communicable diseases; diarrhoeal diseases, dengue hemorrhagic fever, malaria and viral hepatitis headed the list. Nutrition, maternal and child health, environmental health and mental health were foremost among the noncommunicable diseases. There was a discernible shift towards noncommunicable diseases in later years. Studies of other important health-related problems were also supported, including health manpower, nursing and traditional medicine. Of the types of research supported, epidemiological and clinical studies and health system research predominated (i.e. there was little basic research).

Among the research projects supported by the regional office during the three decades of the SEA/ACHR, the regional collaborative study on drug-resistant malaria and the research study on dengue haemorrhagic fever stand out because of their greatly beneficial impact on these major health threats in WHO's South-East Asia and Western Pacific regions. These two regional research projects are of great practical importance, providing tools and methods for monitoring, diagnosing and treating the diseases and also giving insight into patho-physiological mechanisms. The projects also highlighted the regional office's efforts in priority research areas, revealed successes and failures, and brought up important strategic and operational issues with respect to the scientific as well as research management aspects of the WHO programme in the region. The stimulus extended far beyond the actual research projects supported. The catalytic effect is a major accomplishment.

The regional collaborative study on drug-resistant malaria mapped the geographical distribution and degree of resistance to drugs and drug regimes being used in South-East Asian countries at that time and identified alternative, emerging drugs and drug regimes that were effective. This had a tremendous lasting impact on the malaria control programme in all endemic countries of the region and influenced the strategic and operational policies for malaria control, treatment and drug policy.

The regional research programme on dengue haemorrhagic fever comprises several components. One is the project for development of a dengue vaccine. Launched in 1980. the project was undertaken by scientists at Mahidol University (Bangkok) and was supported by the regional office, the government of Thailand and other partners. Its aim was to produce a safe, live, attenuated, immunogenic vaccine against all four strains of the dengue virus. In 1992 WHO announced that the aim had been achieved and the project was successfully concluded. However, a major setback occurred when it was discovered later that some components of the tetravalent vaccine were not sufficiently immunogenic and required further modifications. This is now being followed up by Mahidol University (Bangkok) scientists).

In addition to work on this project, there have also been clinical studies, immunopathological studies, epidemiology and human behaviour studies. These have led to a better knowledge and understanding of the epidemiology, clinical features and immunopathology of dengue haemorrhage fever. Clinical research contributed significantly to improved case management and the reduction in case fatality and mortality rates. However, morbidity remained high and research aimed at reducing morbidity encountered setbacks in the several approaches used – development of a dengue vaccine, studies aimed at identifying epidemiological characteristics of endemic and "silent" areas/countries, and human behaviour research to identify factors that will improve disease control.

Promotion and support of research to facilitate rapid application of knowledge played an important role in the development and understanding of the concept of health systems research and its acceptance by countries. Several interrelated strategies were pursued, namely:

— institutionalization of health systems research;
— direct support for health systems research projects in countries;
— development of WHO collaborating centres on health systems research;
— linkages and integration of health systems research into WHO's technical programmes.

6.4.4 *The role of SEA/ACHR today and in the future*

Most countries in the region have been weaned from dependence on WHO's support, apart from a few of the smaller countries. Since 1976, WHO has built up the research capacities, expertise and experience of countries. Partly because of this, but largely due to their own efforts, most countries are now increasingly self-reliant in research – especially in health systems research, epidemiological research, and clinical research essential for their needs. Some have also conducted research in biotechnology. This in itself can be regarded as one of the major achievements of WHO's collaborative efforts over the years.

WHO's role in promoting, conducting, supporting and coordinating health research in most countries of the region is now minimal. It is limited to advocacy, drawing attention to emerging regional health research needs and opportunities, and promoting and enabling interaction and partnership between scientists and institutions in the region and worldwide.

In the new international health setting of globalization with widening partnerships in which WHO now operates, the function of SEA/ACHR has changed considerably since 1976. Although there is no formal change of the terms of reference, the advice sought from the committee by the regional office has become circumscribed since research capability strengthening activities and research project support are no longer undertaken or have become minimal. Most advice sought concerns research management systems in countries. Increasingly, SEA/ACHR is called upon to advise the regional office on how to support countries to mobilize and utilize the large variety of bilateral and multilateral resources from agencies and developmental groups on health development (each with its own mission, objectives and agenda) in a way that is in accordance with countries' own national health research development aims.

6.5 WHO WESTERN PACIFIC REGION

6.5.1 Introduction

The WHO Western Pacific Region is one of the most diverse of the WHO regions and has rapidly changing economic, political and cultural environments, health systems and health statuses. The Regional Committee, the governing body of WHO in the region and composed of representatives of all 27 Member States, formulates policies of a regional character and reviews the programmes and activities of the WHO Regional Office for the Western Pacific.

6.5.2 History of the Western Pacific Advisory Committee on Medical/Health Research

When established in 1976, the Western Pacific Advisory Committee on Medical Research (WPACMR), like the advisory committees in the other WHO regions, had terms of reference with the following objectives:

- definition of policies for promotion of research in the region;
- determination of regional priorities for research;
- coordination of research between WHO headquarters and regional offices, between regional offices and Member States, and between Member States themselves;
- development of research capability in the region;
- establishment of meaningful collaboration between the WPACMR and the global ACMR;
- establishment of close contact between national and international bodies engaged in research, including assistance in setting up national health research councils or analogous bodies;
- collection of data on institutions, facilities, personnel and projects in the region with a view to developing a regional research information system;
- the stimulation of research in priority areas, improvement of coordination between countries, and promotion and communication between the scientists and institutions working on common problems;
- evaluation of programmes in terms of stated objectives and the mechanisms for implementation.

The WPACMR (or the Western Pacific Advisory Committee on Health Research, or WPACHR, as it was known after 1988), through its recommendations to the WHO Regional Office for the Western Pacific, supported the work conducted by WHO staff in the regional office and in headquarters. Other achievements include:

- recognition of the important role played by research councils and analogous bodies in the development of robust national health research systems in the Member States;
- support given to WHO's special programmes, collaborating centres and research training courses;
- development of a strategic plan for health research (1996) and a strategic

framework for health research (2004);
— engagement of Member States in WHO's global and regional activities (e.g. the Evidence Informed Policy Network (EVIPNet);
— alignment of the regional research agenda with the global agenda using WHO's strategies;
— significant growth in capacity for health research and in the amount of research being conducted in the majority of Member States.

Frequency of committee meetings has varied from annual to biannual (current). This has an impact on what the committee can achieve as to date it has been difficult to engage members between meetings. Continuity of membership (and of the chair) has been important as the committee has sought to add value to its work.

It is also of interest that the majority of the issues discussed at the time the WPACMR was established in the 1970s (e.g. identification of priorities, need to build research capacity, and strengthening of research capability in Member States) are those which continue to engage the WPACHR, Western Pacific Member States and their research communities today.

Lack of resources for the committee or for regional office-initiated research-related activities has been an ongoing concern and has hampered implementation of major regional initiatives such as the strategic framework. Lack of joint meetings with the SEA/ACHR has been a missed opportunity (only a single meeting being held in 1984).

6.5.3 Health research councils and analogous bodies

At the earliest meetings of the WPACMR in the 1970s it was recognized that one of the roles of WHO with respect to health research was to work with national and regional organizations. Coordination of health research within countries and technical cooperation between countries has been a priority for the region and the WPACMR/WPACHR since that time.

Whereas in the early 1950s the region had only two health research councils (in Australia and New Zealand), the past 30 years have seen the development of health research councils or analogous bodies, or at least a focal point for health research in all but the smallest of the Pacific Island countries of the 27 Member States of the WHO Western Pacific Region. In some countries (e.g. China, Fiji, Japan, Lao People's Democratic Republic, Republic of Korea, Malaysia, Mongolia, Papua New Guinea, Philippines, Singapore) excellent progress has been made. Progress in building and/or strengthening national health research systems in other Member States of the region has been slow but steady, and is ongoing.

During this time and under the leadership of four regional directors, the representatives of health research councils or similar bodies have played an increasingly important role in the work of the WPACHR. Originally meeting on their own, then jointly with WPACHR, they are now represented on the WPACHR. The role of the councils has been significant in the development of research policy, funding and management of research, and training of researchers, together with input into regulatory activities such as ethics and dissemination of research findings to policy-makers.

The national health research council and analogous bodies have played an important role as the link between the research community and government and they thus bring valuable perspectives on strategy and research capacity strengthening to the WPACHR. Looking to the future it will be important for these councils in the 27 Member States to establish a regional network and to collaborate with global ACHR initiatives and with similar councils in other regions – especially the WHO South-East Asia Region.

6.5.4 The Institute for Medical Research, Kuala Lumpur, as the WHO Regional Centre for Research and Training in Tropical Diseases and Nutrition

In 1978 WHO made the landmark decision to designate the Institute for Medical Research (IMR) in Kuala Lumpur, Malaysia, as its Regional Centre for Research and Training in Tropical Diseases and Nutrition. As Regional Centre, the IMR's objectives were:

— to develop, through biomedical research, new methods for the diagnosis, treatment and prevention of the major communicable diseases, with special emphasis on the parasitic diseases prevailing in the region;
— to train scientists and technicians in the proper conduct of research for the control of these diseases;
— to act as focal point for the coordination of research and training in the region.

Once the decision was taken, efforts were made to integrate the IMR quickly into the mainstream activities of the WHO Regional Office for the Western Pacific and of TDR which was based at WHO headquarters in Geneva. This was done through a combination of infrastructure support (in terms of equipment and technology) and the posting of consultants in strategic areas, running *pari passu* with staff development activities achieved through the awarding of both short-term and long-term fellowships for training and research grants. In determining the priority areas for support, situational analyses allowed gaps to be identified which needed specific strengthening in terms of capacity and capability. As capability increased, research strengthening grants gave way to competitive research. The inverse relationship between the numbers of these two grants illustrates the acquisition of capacity to compete and be self-reliant.

With these inputs and together with its traditional strengths, the IMR was ready to play its role in devolving its capabilities to other countries in the region. This was initially primarily in training activities through courses in epidemiology and biostatistics for scientists from the countries both at the IMR (35 courses) and in their home countries (9 courses).

Additionally, the Regional Centre was able to synergistically utilize the contributions and inputs from a number of national, regional and international partnerships. As the centre became self-reliant and also more involved with its own national agenda, and as the other countries of the region also began to increase their capacities, WHO support for the centre tapered off. However, the IMR remains designated as the WHO Regional Centre and continues to play an advisory role.

6.5.5 WHO collaborating centres

The Laboratory of Microbiology and Pathology of the Department of Health, Brisbane, Australia, was the first institution in the region to be designated as a collaborating centre. It was named in 1957 as the WHO Collaborating Centre for Reference and Research on Leptospirosis and is still active today.

The number of centres sharply increased after 1980, reaching 165 centres by 1994. There were two main reasons for this: the recognition and designation of many institutions in China and the decentralization of the Research Policy and Cooperation programme at regional level which resulted in an increased need for support from national collaborating institutions. In 2009 there were 194 centres in 10 countries. Three countries host 77% of the collaborating centres in the region (China with 71, Australia with 46 and Japan with 33). The programmes with the largest number of centres are Noncommunicable Diseases with 24, Mental Health and Control of Substance Abuse with 19, and Reproductive Health with 18. Since 1988, national meetings for the directors of all regional WHO collaborating centres have been held in China (at least 9), Malaysia (annually since 1993) and twice each in Australia, Japan and the Republic of Korea. In China, meetings have also been held for all centres in a specific discipline (e.g. primary health care, mental health/neurosciences, and occupational health). In addition, representatives of all collaborating centres in Shanghai have met at least five times. Each centre must submit an annual report immediately after the end of each year. This report covers only the activities of the institution as a WHO collaborating centre and reflects the progress made by the centre. It was noted that many were unaware of the existence of other centres in the region or even in their own countries, despite being involved in similar programmes of work.

6.5.6 The future

Historically, one of WHO's greatest strengths has been its ability to adapt to evolving circumstances, as exemplified by health priorities being adjusted from time to time. In this regard, the members of the WPACHR, the health research councils or analogous bodies, and the regional advisors of technical units will continue to be involved in identifying the priorities in health research within this region. Continued efforts will be made to strengthen the research capabilities in the region by means of providing research grants, research training awards at scientific, technological and managerial levels, and national workshops on research design and methodology. Technical units will be encouraged to initiate commissioned research in the priority areas. In addition, countries will be encouraged and supported to initiate operational research in priority areas. Research promotion activities should continue to be directed to less developed countries such as Cambodia, Lao People's Democratic Republic, Mongolia, Pacific island countries and Viet Nam. In order to look for effective ways to use the increasingly limited resources, the WHO collaborating centres should be encouraged to work together with WHO and among themselves to develop and support work in the priority areas identified by WHO. One of the most challenging tasks for the regional office will be to continue to increase the involvement of all collaborating centres. To offset the limited research budget of the Research Policy and Cooperation programme in the regional office, efforts must continue to obtain funds from extrabudgetary sources.

6.6 PAN AMERICAN HEALTH ORGANIZATION

6.6.1 Introduction

In 1962, the Pan American Health Organization (PAHO), WHO's Regional Office for the Americas, established its Advisory Committee on Medical Research (ACMR) "to review existing and proposed research programmes and make appropriate suggestions" and "to recommend the basis for a long-term research policy for present and future projects, to be approved by the Governing Bodies of the Pan American Health Organization". In 1986, the committee changed its name to the Advisory Committee for Health Research (ACHR). The next sections highlight a number of key contributions since the committee's creation.

6.6.2 Strengthening "good" governance and stewardship for research and the national health research systems in Latin American and Caribbean countries

Stimulating biomedical research

The ACMR's responsibilities included the examination and stimulation of the biomedical research fields that dealt with the organization's objectives, and the formulation of opinions on policy related to research, training and education. Following ACMR's recommendation, in 1962 the XVI Pan American Sanitary Conference established research as a major item in PAHO's policy; the policy statements stressed the organization's role in assisting countries to develop the necessary research resources.

In 1964, PAHO's governing bodies approved a list of 45 projects to be developed with scientists and institutions from all over the Americas, and the committee suggested that various standardized protocols be developed on such topics as tuberculosis programmes and protection against radiation.

By 1965, ACMR expressed concern about several issues: the uneven distribution of research efforts in the Americas, limited tradition in science in Latin American and Caribbean countries, weaknesses in research on clinical investigation epidemiology, virology, and public health administration, a lack of resources in many countries, the structural rigidity of universities and poor scientific communication. The committee focused on educational research as a way to maintain quality standards of scientists and doctors in training and to address the trend in Latin America and the Caribbean for them to leave their countries of origin in pursuit of work opportunities elsewhere, especially in the United States.

In the 1967 Declaration by the Presidents of the Americas at Punta del Este, Uruguay, the heads of state urged that a regional programme be put in place to foster scientific and technological development. For the first time in Latin America's history, presidents had concurred on funding science and technology. Recommendations were made for including selected fields, including basic sciences, biochemistry, physiology, genetics and microbiology.

Formulating research policy

In the first 15 years of the ACMR's operation, recommendations focused on stimulating and supporting biomedical research and research training. There was emphasis on collaborative multinational projects, the strengthening of biomedical communications and resources through scientific meetings and the provision of access to scientific production and other resources, and the promotion and application of operations research to improve the efficiency of health facilities and programmes. Many experts became consultants to the committee, and 216 technical reports and 31 scientific monographs were published. PAHO had to align its priorities with those of granting agencies, and the organization contributed 30% of the ACHR's budget. The Office of Research Coordination implemented the Organization's policy by identifying research problems and opportunities, particularly regarding projects suited for multicountry collaboration efforts, and by exploring options for acquiring financial support from granting agencies.

Although in 1962 most Latin American and Caribbean countries lacked functional scientific or technological infrastructures, by the mid 1980s most of them had established institutions and systems to promote and support science and technology activities. In stressing the importance of biotechnology, ACHR gave priority to biotechnological research geared to producing vaccines and developing diagnostic methods, and developing insecticides and drugs. Member countries were encouraged to include the development and strengthening of biotechnology in their national policies on science and technology for economic and social development, and for these purposes, contacts were established with the government agencies and research councils in charge of planning and supporting developmental and technological research in member countries.

In 1985, PAHO's Research Grants Programme became a technical cooperation mechanism designed to generate knowledge that could address priority health issues; subcommittees of the ACMR (renamed the Advisory Committee on Health Research, or ACHR, in 1986) were created to focus on biotechnology and health systems research.

By the mid-1990s, the ACHR focused on orienting PAHO's research policies, along with other technical cooperation activities of the organization, to concentrate its activities on five areas selected by the governing bodies according to PAHO's 1995–1998 strategic and programmatic orientations.

By the mid-1990s PAHO's research areas were:

— health and development;
— health promotion and protection;
— health systems development;
— environmental protection and development;
— disease prevention and control.

Beginning in 1995, PAHO's Director (in that year, Dr. George A. O. Alleyne) guided the execution of the organization's regional programming, reflecting persistent intentions to seek equity and "Pan Americanism". The ACHR recommended that clear and formal criteria and mechanisms for reviewing projects be established, involving many

PAHO divisions, Pan American centres and country offices. PAHOs Regional Programme of Bioethics analysed the ethical implications of research and formulated standards relating to new trends, such as the commercialization of knowledge and the gene pool. Bioethics and the ethical regulation of research became a cornerstone in the development of health research systems. In 1997, particular attention was paid to topics such as "the privatization of knowledge and the strengthening of mechanisms for controlling intellectual property and its impact on health research in the Region".

6.6.3 Health research promotion and the common good

During the 1960s, PAHO's research programme played an important role in stimulating and strengthening the resources and capabilities for biomedical research in the Americas. These efforts resulted in the development of research projects in a wide range of fields: 1001 projects were sponsored, supported and/or carried out by PAHO between 1961 and 1983. Of these, 32% were related to zoonoses and foot-and-mouth disease, 14% to food and nutrition, 10% to infectious diseases, 25% to environmental health, parasitic and chronic diseases, and perinatology, with the remaining projects (19%) covering other public health topics. PAHO staff conducted 634 of these projects, and 367 were carried out by local researchers. A more comprehensive scrutiny of PAHO's research activities requires a consideration of all research- related technical cooperation activities, such as those related to health promotion and the provision of advisory services and information. For instance, 7% of the 5703 technical cooperation activities programmed for 1984 were considered to be research activities, and technical cooperation in the area of research accounted for 17% of all activities programmed in the countries. There have been significant variations in the PAHO budget devoted to research. However, establishing how much has been invested in research has been a challenge because resources for research are not exclusively channelled through the Research Promotion and Development division. Most resources are channelled through country offices, technical teams and PAHO centres.

When classified by functional approach, the allocation of resources by biennial programme budget showed that, for the 1998–1999 biennium, regional programmes devoted three times more for research promotion than country offices did. Yet only 6% of the total operational budget was allocated for this functional approach. Furthermore, using the same classification, the amount allocated in the same biennium was half that allocated in 1990.

During the late 1980s, PAHO began using functional approaches as a way to differentiate the types of technical cooperation provided to countries. Such classification complemented the organization's efforts to develop a workplan tailored to the needs of its members. Six functional approaches were identified, namely: resource mobilization; information dissemination; training; norms, plans and policies; research promotion; and direct technical cooperation.

A study on research proposals considered by the PAHO governing bodies during the 1942–1984 period found that about one third of the proposals addressed communicable diseases, 21% the planning and administration of health services, and the remaining

49% was divided among work in the areas of chronic diseases, nutrition, environmental health, maternal and child health, material resources, and other health programmes. Several indicators for research and development in Latin America and the Caribbean improved during the 1990s, as compared to the 1980s, and expenditure increased by 56% between 1990 and 1996 in Argentina, Brazil and Mexico.

Beginning in 1969 and spanning more than four decades, the Instituto de Nutrición de Centro América y Panama (INCAP) has conducted a series of longitudinal and follow-up studies. This research assesses the effects of intrauterine and preschool nutrition on growth, development and human capital formation, and has also focused on the following areas: physical development, medical history and cardiovascular risk, schooling attainment and cognitive functioning, occupational income and wealth, mother-child interaction, and diet and physical activity. This study has resulted in more than 200 publications influencing knowledge about the impact of early life nutrition on a variety of key aspects of human development.

6.6.4 Improving competencies for health research

The training of human resources for health research grew considerably during the final two decades of the 20th century in Latin America and the Caribbean. Fellowships for doctoral programmes abroad began to receive substantial financial support from the public sector through national councils of science and technology, and through loans from diverse entities. Favourable conditions were created in such Member States as Argentina, Brazil, Chile, Colombia, Mexico and Venezuela to develop doctoral-level national research training programmes. Countries began to develop partnerships and agreements to establish cooperative programmes and to integrate doctorate studies utilizing the expertise of local academic and research institutions.

To stimulate the production of scientific literature, the Fred L. Soper Award for Excellence in Health Literature was created in 1990 as a result of a partnership between the Pan American Health and Education Foundation (PAHEF) and PAHO. Similarly, to stimulate the strengthening of capacities for bioethical analysis among young researchers, the Secretary of Health of Mexico, PAHEF and PAHO partnered to create the Manuel Velasco-Suárez Award in Bioethics in 2002. Recipients of these awards are given a cash prize and a certificate of recognition in a special PAHO ceremony.

6.6.5 Developing and maintaining sustainable health research systems

Examples of direct accomplishments of PAHO (and WHO), under the guidance of the ACHR, are the 189 successful collaborating centres/programmes established in Latin America and the Caribbean (http://www.bireme.br/whocc/). The WHO collaborating centres include research institutes, parts of universities or academic centres that carry out activities in support of the organization's programmes on areas such as nursing, occupational health, communicable diseases, nutrition, mental health, chronic diseases and health technologies.

In 1966, the 19th World Health Assembly requested the WHO Director-General to initiate action to achieve a worldwide smallpox eradication programme that included producing the vaccine, training technicians, providing essential supplies, and organizing programmes in the countries. Historically, the eradication of smallpox remains one of the greatest achievements of WHO: in 1980, the Thirty-third World Health Assembly endorsed the conclusions of the Global Commission for the Certification of Smallpox Eradication (confirming that smallpox had been eradicated). Previously, in 1973, the XXII PAHO Directing Council had declared the disease eradicated from the Americas, making this region the first to achieve this status.

In 1985, PAHO proposed interrupting the transmission of wild poliovirus in the western hemisphere by 1990; the proposal was endorsed by all Member States and supported by key international partner agencies and organizations. The organization sponsored international research, collaborated in trials of live attenuated poliovirus vaccine, assisted in organizing vaccination programmes and supported the supply of vaccines and equipment. In 1994 the International Commission for the Certification of Poliomyelitis Eradication in the Americas announced that wild poliovirus transmission had been interrupted in the Americas.

A programme for the eradication in the Americas of *Aedes aegypti*, the mosquito vector of both yellow fever and dengue, was planned and initiated by PAHO in 1946. Substantial progress was made, and several countries were able to eradicate this mosquito and stayed *Aedes aegypti*-free from 1961 to 1974. However, some countries gradually became reinfested over time, and the increasing occurrence of dengue fever and dengue hemorrhagic fever epidemics during the 1990s revealed a setback in the goal of achieving eradication. PAHO, through its Regional Programme on Tuberculosis, prepared a hemisphere-wide plan to combat this disease and, by 1973, mortality from tuberculosis significantly dropped compared with 1953 rates as reported in the History of the Pan American Health Organization (see: http://www.pitt.edu/~super1/lecture/lec0291/fulltext.htm).

The ACMR recommended programmes and collaborative studies on maternal and child health and disease prevention, to plan and implement immunization programmes, to promote breastfeeding and health education of mothers, and to strengthen prenatal and perinatal health services programmes. Since its earliest days, the ACMR has endorsed strategies to increase access to clean drinking water and provide adequate sanitation services for the region's underserved populations and has encouraged the production of needed research in this area. PAHO has provided technical cooperation to Member States to support basic sanitation infrastructure and services and, on an ongoing basis, studies the determinants of unequal distribution among countries and geographical regions within countries, and between urban and rural settings. By 2002 about 11% of the population of Latin America and the Caribbean remained without access to safe water and 25% lacked access to basic sanitation (*37*). The latest (2010) WHO/UNICEF report confirms that advances continue to be made towards greater access to safe drinking-water; however, about 7% of the population of LAC remained without access to safe water and 20% lacked access to basic sanitation in 2008 (*38*). Yet the implementation of water and sanitation programmes, alongside those aiming to reduce the spread of diseases and control of diarrheal diseases, has led to a decrease in infant mortality in Latin America and the Caribbean. Another major achievement of PAHO was through its "Inter-American Investigation of Mortality" research project conducted during the 1960s that collected information on some 35,000 child mortality cases. The database provided input for the development of child mortality prevention projects and further research, which ultimately resulted in a reduction in childhood deaths.

During the 1960s, INCAP research developed *Incaparina*, a low-cost, high-protein dietary supplement based on cottonseed flour, or soya and vegetables, and enriched with vitamins and minerals, and initiated its mass production in Central America. Activities to reduce chronic malnutrition have been successful in this subregion, largely due to PAHO's efforts to provide technical cooperation, mobilize resources, and transfer technologies and methodologies to national institutions. Through its Regional Programme on Disability Prevention and Rehabilitation, PAHO has provided technical cooperation to Member States for the generation of policies, plans, interventions and projects to prevent disability and to enable the rehabilitation of disabled people. With the participation of PAHO/WHO collaborating centres, various countries have adopted surveillance systems for occupational accidents. In 2005, participants in the Ibero-American Summit held in Salamanca, Spain, approved the creation of four Ibero-American health cooperation networks: the Donation and Transplant Network, coordinated by Spain, the Public Health Teaching and Research Network, coordinated by Costa Rica, the Tobacco Control Network, coordinated by Brazil and the Drug Policy Network, coordinated by Argentina.

6.6.6 *Health research alliances and collaboration*

From its creation, the ACMR (and later, the ACHR) has stressed the importance of catalyzing the development and strengthening of strategic partnerships to advance health research. Since 1962, PAHO has received invaluable support from an important number of organizations, agencies, institutions and individuals.

The U.S. National Institutes of Health (NIH), for instance, provided a grant for PAHO to establish the Office of Research Coordination (currently the Research Promotion and Development team) and the organization received substantial support from grant agencies, among which the NIH/U.S. Public Health Service figured most prominently during the early 1960s. The ACMR recommended that the regional reference centre, Adolfo Lutz Institute, collaborate with the regional reference centre at the U.S. Centres for Disease Control and Prevention in Atlanta, Georgia. The Caribbean Food and Nutrition Institute began operation as a collaborative project between PAHO, the Food and Agriculture Organization of the United Nations, the University of West Indies, and the governments of Jamaica and Trinidad and Tobago, with support from the William Waterman Fund. An agreement with Milbank Memorial Fund for a programme for rational development of human resources for health in the Caribbean and cooperation with Brazilian libraries and the biomedical community became part of these strategic partnerships developed upon recommendations issued by the ACMR.

The NIH sponsored research on computer applications in the life sciences. In the mid-1970s, the U.S. National Library of Medicine announced plans for testing the MEDLINE system in Brazil and establishing an audiovisual centre at the PAHO Regional Library of Medicine (today known as the Latin American and Caribbean Centre on Health Sciences Information, or BIREME) with funds from the United Nations Development Programme (UNDP), the Government of Brazil and the State of São Paulo. Funds were provided to PAHO by the Rockefeller Foundation for the Regional Vaccine System (SIREVA), which was launched in 1994 to promote a regional quality control network and certification system.

In addition to supporting research projects in the Americas, TDR has collaborated with PAHO/WHO collaborating centres in the implementation of a "train-the-trainers" scheme to develop sustainable research project management skills in PAHO Member States.

The "Convergence Project" should also be mentioned as an interagency initiative aimed at promoting technical cooperation among developing countries for the creation of projects and programmes in the area of the health sciences and technology. Its partners include the Latin American Economic System, UNDP, the Economic Commission for Latin America and the Caribbean, the United Nations Educational, Scientific and Cultural Organization, and PAHO.

Over the last three decades, the nations of the Caribbean Community (CARICOM) have established five regional health institutions: the Caribbean Epidemiology Centre, the Caribbean Food and Nutrition Institute, the Caribbean Environmental Health Institute, the Caribbean Health Research Council and the Caribbean Regional Drug-testing Laboratory.

The Programme for Research and Training in Public Health was established with the Carlos III Institute of Health in Madrid, Spain, through an agreement signed by PAHO and the Government of Spain. The Latin American Biological Network and PAHO signed an agreement to finance biomedical research projects of interest to public health; an additional agreement between the International Clearinghouse for the Health Sector Reform Initiative (ICHSRI/NADIR) and PAHO was also signed to support research on sectoral reforms and their effects, access to health services, and their financing and utilization in developing countries.

To promote broader participation of society in research, partnerships have been forged to make novel educational resources available to the public.

6.6.7 Conclusion

Throughout the ACHR's life, the research and health landscapes have changed dramatically. For instance, significant progress has been attained in eradicating infectious diseases (e.g. polio has been eradicated from all countries in the Americas) and non-communicable diseases, research capabilities and production have increased exponentially, access to evidence from research has greatly improved with the arrival of new information and communication technologies, such as the Internet, and new methodologies have been developed to summarize information and deliver it in formats that address the needs of different audiences. Yet, new challenges continue to emerge and health improvement goals are always changing. As conditions improve, new goals are set to address emerging challenges, maintain achievements and improve equity. Research as a public health function still needs to be strengthened in many countries and international agendas dealing with the production and implementation of knowledge were proposed at milestone events such as the 2004 Ministerial Summit on Health Research. WHO's endorsement of the recommendations issued at such events has been followed by proposals and actions that are being implemented. On all these fronts, the ACHR has been extraordinarily helpful to PAHO and it remains relevant for addressing the challenges PAHO must face in the 21st century. The ACHR's guidance will continue to be essential for building the future of health and health research in Latin American and Caribbean countries.

7. Epilogue

Although it has often been argued that WHO is not a research organization, it is clear that the organization is managing a knowledge-based programme of work. Science and research are part and parcel of all its technical activities. Furthermore, multidisciplinarity is a hallmark of all these efforts, particularly when the translation and application of knowledge are required at local level.

This overview has documented how WHO was equipped both at the conceptual and operational levels to cope with the difficult and challenging problems of world health as well as the various types of research needed to alleviate them.

To quote a prominent member of the (global) Advisory Committee on Medical Research:

> "I challenge the oft-repeated statement that what is needed in the under-developed, economically underdeveloped societies in medicine and health, is the application of what we know now – I claim we do not know it now and that our current biomedical technology has been Darwinianly adapted to the problems of an industrialized society which it has started not to fit- and that the problems of the overly-traditional societies are of a quite different nature and require the development of new knowledge before we can successfully meet them…"

(Prof.W.Mc Dermott, ACMR, 1967)

8. WHO Research for Health Strategy approved by the Sixty-third World Health Assembly 2010

May 2010 saw the first organization-wide strategy on research approved by the World Health Assembly within Resolution WHA63.21. The Resolution sets out WHO's role and responsibilities in health research in the WHO strategy on research for health, Sixty-third World Health Assembly paper A63.22. The strategy is organized around five main goals:

Capacity – building capacity to strengthen health research systems.

Priorities – supporting the setting of research priorities that meet health needs particularly in low and middle income countries.

Standards – creating an environment to create good research practice and enable the greater sharing of research evidence, tools and materials.

Translation – ensuring quality evidence is turned into products and policy.

Organization – action to strengthen the research culture within WHO and improve the management and coordination of WHO research activities.

References

(Items marked (*) are available through the WHO Library Information Service online database WHOLIS at http://dosei.who.int)

(1) (*) WHO. *The Advisory Committee on Health Research: an overview.* Technical document WHO/RPS/ACHR/97.1. Geneva, World Health Organization, 1997 (http://whqlibdoc.who.int/hq/1997/WHO_RPS_ACHR_97.1.pdf, accessed 29 Sept. 2010).

(2) Mansourian B. *Research in the World Health Organization: fifty years of progress.* Lecture at the Royal Academy of Overseas Sciences, Brussels, 25 February 2003.

(3) WHO. *The third ten years of the World Health Organization, 1968–1977.* Geneva, World Health Organization, 2009.

(4) Commission on Health Research for Health Development. *Health research: essential link to equity in development.* New York, NY, Oxford University Press, 1990.

(5) Davies M, Mansourian B. *Research strategies for health.* Lewiston, NY, and Toronto, Hogrefe and Huber, 1992 [Proceedings of a conference on research, under the auspices of the World Health Assembly].

(6) COHRED. *Essential national health research and priority setting: lessons learned.* Document 97.3. Geneva, Council on Health Research for Development, 1997.

(7) World Bank. *World development report 1993: investing in health.* New York, NY, Oxford University Press, 1993.

(8) Murray CJL, Lopez A, eds. *The global burden of disease.* Cambridge, MA, Harvard University Press, 1996.

(9) WHO. *Investing in health research and development. Report of the Ad Hoc Committee on Health Research relating to future intervention options.* Geneva, World Health Organization, 1996.

(10) Web site of the Global Forum for Health Research at www.globalforumhealth.org.

(11) (*) WHO. Reports of the Advisory Committee on Medical Research and the Advisory Committee on Health Research (all reports).

(12) (*) WHO. *Health research strategy for Health for All by the Year 2000. Report of a subcommittee of the ACHR.* Technical document WHO/RPD/ACHR(HRS)/86. Geneva, World Health Organization, 1986.

(13) (*) WHO. *Enhancement of transfer of technology to developing countries with special reference to health. Report of a subcommittee of the ACHR.* Technical document WHO/RPD/ACHR(TT)/87. Geneva, World Health Organization, 1987 (http://whqlibdoc.who.int/hq/1987/WHO_RPD_ACHR(TT)_87.pdf, accessed 29 Sept. 2010).

(14) (*) WHO. *Enhancement of transfer of technology to developing countries with special reference to health: technology transfer in prosthetics and orthotics for the developing world.* Geneva, World Health Organization, 1986.

(15) (*) WHO. *Enhancement of transfer of technology to developing countries with special reference to health: new materials and developments in materials technology.* Geneva, World Health Organization, 1986.

(16) (*) WHO. *Enhancement of transfer of technology to developing countries with special reference to health: biosensors in primary health care.* Geneva, World Health Organization, 1986.

(17) (*) WHO. *Enhancement of transfer of technology to developing countries with special reference to health: information and systems science.* Geneva, World Health Organization, 1986.

(18) (*) WHO. *Research for health: principles, perspectives and strategies.* Technical document WHO/RPD/ACHR(HRS)/93. Geneva, World Health Organization, 1993 (http://whqlibdoc.who.int/hq/1993/WHO_RPD_ACHR_(HRS)_93.pdf, accessed 29 Sept. 2010).

(19) (*) WHO. *A research policy agenda for science and technology to support global health development.* Technical document WHO/RPS/ACHR/98.1. Geneva, World Health Organization, 1998 (http://whqlibdoc.who.int/hq/1998/WHO_RPS_ACHR_98.1.pdf, accessed 29 Sept. 2010).

(20) Black D. Priorities in biomedical research: indices of burden. *British Medical Journal of Preventive and Social Medicine*, 1975, 89(4).

(21) Patel M. An economic evaluation of Health for All. *Health Policy and Planning*, 1986, 1(1):37–47.

(22) *The role of health research in the strategy for Health for All by the year 2000.* Background document for technical discussions at the World Health Assembly, May 1990. Geneva, World Health Organization, 1990.

(23) Kaplan M. Science's role in the World Health Organization. *Science*, 1973, 180(4090):1028.

(24) (*) Manciaux M. *The WHO collaborating centres: an analytical review.* Technical document WHO/RPS/ACHR/98.4. Geneva, World Health Organization, 1998 (http://whqlibdoc.who.int/hq/1998/WHO_RPS_ACHR_98.4.pdf, accessed 29 Sept. 2010).

(25) PAHO. *Pan American Centers. Report of a study group.* Document CSP20/3 presented to the XX Pan American Sanitary Conference, 30th Americas Regional Committee meeting, St George's, Grenada, September 1978 (http://hist.library.paho.org/English/GOV/CSP/20_3.pdf, accessed 29 Sept. 2010).

(26) Lederberg J. Medical science, infectious disease and the unity of humankind. *Journal of the American Medical Association*, 1988, 260(5):684–685.

(27) Cvjetanovic Grab B, Uemura K. Epidemiological model of typhoid fever and its use in the planning and evaluation of antityphoid immunization and sanitation programmes. *Bulletin of the World Health Organization*, 1971, 45:53–75.

(28) Feldstein MS, Piot MA, Sundaresan TK. Resource allocation model for public health planning, a case study of tuberculosis control. *Bulletin of the World Health Organization*, 1973, 48(Supplement).

(29) Mansourian BG, Sayers BMcA. Pattern analysis in the study of infantile disease and other epidemiological problems. *Bulletin of the World Health Organization*, 1979, 57:865–885.

(30) WHO. *Research methods for health development*. Technical document RPD/SOC/85. Geneva, World Health Organization, 1985.

(31) Mansourian PG. *The prospects of automation from the viewpoint of the World Health Organization*. In: Automation in microbiology and immunology. Proceedings of a conference, 3–6 June 1973, Stockholm. New York and London, John Wiley & sons, 1975.

(32) Mott KE, Nuttall I, Desjeux P, Cottand P. New geographical approaches to control of some parasitic zoonoses. *Bulletin of the World Health Organization*, 1995,73(2):247–257.

(33) Nuttall I, O'Neill K, Meert J-P. Systèmes d'information géographique et lutte contre les maladies tropicales. *Médecine Tropicale*, 1998, 58:3.

(34) Mansourian PG, Sayers McA, Newell KW, Tan TP. A pattern analysis study of weanling diarrhoeal disease of infants. *International Journal of Epidemiology*, 1975, 4(3):173–188.

(35) Sayers B McA, Mansourian BG, Phan Tan T, Bögel K. A pattern analysis study of a wild-life rabies epizootic. *Medical Informatics*, 1977, 2:11–34.

(36) Attinger EO, Ahuja D. Health and socioeconomic change. *IEEE Transactions on Man, Systems and Cybernetics*, 1980, SMC-10(12):781–796.

(37) WHO/UNICEF Joint Monitoring Programme for Water Supply and Sanitation; Meeting the MDG drinking water and sanitation target: a mid-term assessment of progress, 2004

(38) /UNICEF Joint Monitoring Programme for Water Supply and Sanitation. Progress on Sanitation and Drinking-water: 2010 Update.

Further reading

Mahfouz,MM. Research, society and human values. *WHO Chronicle*, 1977, 31:56–59.

Saracci R. What health for whom? A challenge for epidemiology. *World Health Forum*, 1998, 19:3–5 (accessible at http://whqlibdoc.who.int/whf/1998/vol19-no1/WHF_1998_19(1)_p3-5.pdf, accessed 29 Sept. 2010).

Sayers B McA. Knowledge-based technology in the service of health. *World Health Forum*, 1998, 19:15–20. [A discussion of recent methods, based on computational logic for developing indicators.]

Sayers B McA (chair). 1999. *Health assessment: complexities, trends and opportunities*. Geneva, internal World Health Organization document, 83 pp. [A report of a subcommittee of WHO's Advisory Committee on Health Research, on "Measurement of Health".]

Sayers B McA, Ross AJ, Saengcharoenrat P, Mansourian BG. *Pattern analysis of fox rabies case occurrences in Europe*. In: Bacon PJ, ed. Mathematical aspects of rabies. Chichester, Academic Press, 1984.

WHO. *A research policy agenda for science and technology to support global health development: a synopsis*. Geneva, World Health Organization, Advisory Committee on Health Research,1998 (http://whqlibdoc.who.int/hq/1998/WHO_RPS_ACHR_98.1.pdf, accessed 29 Sept. 2010).

WHO. *Excerpt from report of the Subcommittee on Health and the Economy of the WHO Advisory Committee on Health Research*. Document EB89/INF.DOC./8. Geneva, World Health Organization, 1991.

WHO. *Making a Difference*. 30 Years of Research and Capacity Building in Tropical Diseases, 2007

WHO. *Neuroscience, neurology and health*. Geneva, World Health Organization, Advisory Committee on Health Research, 1997.

WHO. *Recent achievements in neurosciences*. Geneva, World Health Organization, Advisory Committee on Health Research, 1998 (http://whqlibdoc.who.int/hq/1998/WHO_RPS_ACHR_98.3.pdf, accessed 29 Sept. 2010).

WHO. *The first ten years of the World Health Organization* (1948–1957). Geneva, World Health Organization, 1958.

WHO. *The second ten years of the World Health Organization* (1958–1967). Geneva, World Health Organization, 1968.

WHO. *Science and technology for health: a newsletter*. Geneva, World Health Organization, Advisory Committee for Health Research.

WHO. *Research on aging: report of a subcommittee of the ACHR*. Geneva, World Health Organization, Office of Research Promotion and Development, 1986.

WHO. *Health manpower research: report of a subcommittee of the ACHR*. Unpublished document ACHR28/86.7,Add.1. Geneva, World Health Organization, Office of Research Promotion and Development, 1986.

WHO. *Report of the ACHR Subcommittee on Health and the Economy*. Geneva, World Health Organization, Advisory Committee on Health Research, 1992.

WHO. *Research policy and strategy: report by the Director-General*. Geneva, World Health Organization, Advisory Committee on Health Research, 1995.

WHO/CIOMS. *The impact of scientific advances on future health: report of a WHO-CIOMS colloquium, Charlottesville, Virginia, 20–24 June 1994*. Document WHO/RPS/ACHR-CIOMS/95. Geneva, World Health Organization and CIOMS, 1995 (http://whqlibdoc.who.int/hq/1995/WHO_RPS_ACHR-CIOMS_95.pdf, accessed 29 Sept. 2010).

Annexes

Annex 1

Summary of the report of the ACMR Subcommittee on the Enhancement of Transfer of Technology to Developing Countries with Special Reference to Health, 1986[1]

The report discusses five major aspect of technology transfer.

A country should decide on its requirements for health-related technology and an early step towards this is the development of a National Health Policy. This should provide a balance between national health goals and resources which should lead to the formulation of priorities. A major requirement is the need for political commitment to achieve these priorities.

Early steps were the establishment of a health infrastructure and the development of a health technology policy. This had two main components – manpower and technology. Their delineation would be facilitated if the health problems of the country could be clearly defined. These problems will differ from country to country, with different emphasis. The technology to be transferred may include procedures, techniques, equipment and facilities for training. The technology transferred should be 'appropriate' i.e. facilitating the provision of health care which is made available or is accessible to everyone in the community and acceptable to all. A wide range of technology is available for transfer but some has major cost implications. Some is highly cost-effective, benefiting many for long periods. Some is palliative, benefiting few for short periods. The latter should not be encouraged at the expense of the former.

Technology transfer by provider countries

Because of different interests of the provider of the technology, the process of technology transfer would have to be tailored to meet the objectives of both the donor and the recipient. Technology transfer could occur by means of donation from one county to another, with or without a linked agreement, by a straight commercial transaction, by a bilateral agreement for joint investment, or by some combination of these mechanisms. The success of the transfer depends on many factors including social, economic, political and trade policies of each partner; the process of technology transfer has to be adjusted for individual situations. The subcommittee recognized the complexity of the process and acknowledged that there is no sure formula for success. There is a need for an independent third party which could help in the formulation of the policy of both partners and in the planning and implementation of the programme as well as to arbitrate in conflicts which may arise; WHO can play a useful role in this respect.

---

[1] For details of the report of the ACMR Subcommittee on the Enhancement of Transfer of Technology to Developing Countries with Special Reference to Health, see ref. 13. The full report is available online at http://whqlibdoc.who.int/hq/1987/WHO_RPD_ACHR(TT)_87.pdf.

The subcommittee discussed the need for 'bridging' mechanisms to facilitate the transfer process. In some countries, the establishment of Research and Development Unit (s) comprising a group of resource personnel would be advantageous. Such a unit would evaluate the technology to be transferred in relation to the needs of the country, it would advise on equipment to be obtained, with emphasis on factors such as design simplicity, reliability, availability of spare parts, ease of maintenance, etc. Such a unit would be based in the user country, not the provider country; in consequence, the developing country would, visibly and concretely, have the responsibility for the choice and use of the transferred technology. The unit would be staffed by trained personnel who could interact with the suppliers of technology at different levels, such as design of equipment, engineering expertise, and awareness of servicing requirements. When necessary, staff might carry out limited studies to test equipment for reliability, etc.

Appropriate technologies based on new scientific concepts

Biological sciences

The subcommittee nominated ten new developments which had great potential in this respect. Most of these were very relevant to three important areas of health care – vaccine development (e.g. analysis of the structure and function of genomes of infectious agents, production of antigens by recombinant DNA technology, etc.), improved techniques for diagnosis (e.g. monoclonal antibodies for the identification of components of infectious agents, and of agents causing epidemics, etc.) and early detection of hereditary disorders (e.g. use of DNA probes to provide a sound basis for genetic advice and for the development of genetic approaches to health promotion, the modulation of gene expression in certain diseases).

These new technologies are also very relevant to existing WHO programmes. Thus, there are four programmes in which the development of new vaccines is a component: **(a)** the Special Programme for Research and Training in Tropical Diseases (TDR); **(b)** the Diarrhoeal Diseases Control Programme (CDD); **(c)** the Special Programme of Research, Development and Research Training in Human Reproduction (HRP), and **(d)** the Vaccine Development Programme.

WHO had made considerable efforts to examine the use of new diagnostic techniques, particularly those based on monoclonal antibodies, for use at the primary health care level and the potential use of nucleic acid probes for diagnosis of hereditary traits and infectious agents.

Physical sciences

There is an extensive range of potentially applicable new technologies in the physical sciences but the subcommittee focused on those with great potential. These are: microelectronics and information technology, from simple solar-powered calculators, hand-held microelectronic devices that display likely diagnoses and suggestions for action, to "expert systems" (mimicking human intelligence) with great potential for the training of health personnel; the use of microprocessor networks for data acquisition as part of a health information system; materials technology and surface science (better water filtration and piping systems, materials with a shape memory, cheap lenses materials, solid state electrolytes leading to better batteries (for solar energy storage); and systems technology and modelling (planning strategies for health care systems, modelling drug development and/or drug delivery systems).

Emerging technologies

The subcommittee noted a number of emerging technologies which were likely to have an increasing impact in the health area. Examples were the use of biosensors in diagnosis (combining biological into physical systems), computer graphics for drug design, lasers and fibre optics in surgery and instrumentation.

It was noted that there could often be significant advantages in combining technologies from both areas and the subcommittee proposed pilot projects which illustrated this.

The contribution of the new technologies to national health programmes

The subcommittee pointed out that new technologies could be applied at all levels of a national health programme which might consist of five sectors: (1) training of personnel, (2) prevention of disease, (3) detection of disease, (4) treatment of disease, and (5) rehabilitation. Examples were given of their application in each of these areas. The subcommittee stressed that many of the technologies were particularly effective in the first three areas which are 'cost-effective'. Thus, recent advances in information technology could have a very great impact at the training level, from surgeons and physicians in medical schools to paramedical workers at the village level. Advanced biotechnology, especially in the provision of safe, stable, cheap and effective vaccines for the control of infectious diseases and of human fertility, has much to offer in the second area. Efficient data collection and processing can warn of incipient epidemics of both communicable and non-communicable diseases. Systems technology can model specific control programmes. In the third area, monoclonal antibodies and nucleic acid probes will become increasingly important over time.

These technologies can also have an impact in the last two areas – e.g. production of chemicals and biologicals for treatment of disease and newer materials for rehabilitation needs.

Roles for WHO

Much of WHO's activities are already concerned with particular aspects of technology transfer. The Special Programmes made particular contributions in this respect. The roles are:

i. to advise on the formulation of a national health technology policy;
ii. to advise the country on the choice of technology to be transferred through appropriate assessment by in-house expertise or on advice from consultants;
iii. to promote the establishment of groups of resource persons in the country with necessary expertise for the related technology;
iv. to facilitate exchange of information and expertise necessary for the implementation of the technology transfer;
v. to identify WHO collaborating centres that could provide appropriate technical and managerial advice;
vi. to further assist in the provision of training of technical staff, through collaborating centres or through agreements with higher technical institutes;
vii. to provide, advice and assist, in an impartial manner, in negotiations between the supplier of the technology and the host country.

Conclusion

Far from being the prerogative of scientists and industries in industrialized countries, the subcommittee is convinced that the transfer of technologies arising from the new scientific discoveries should be vigorously encouraged as they could have a "leapfrogging" effect in enhancing the delivery of improved health care to people in developing countries. The mechanisms proposed in the report are aimed at providing an environment in which the transfer of appropriate technology becomes a partnership so that both countries could benefit; a user country should not be the subject of economic or technological domination by a provider country. Specific pilot projects were proposed by the subcommittee which, if implemented, could act as examples of effective technology transfer.

Annex 2
The Research policy agenda, 1998 (excerpts)[1]

Locating, utilizing and improving existing knowledge

The arrival of the Internet, electronic mail and the World Wide Web has made the exchange of ideas, information, research data and research papers easy, economical and rapid. This is a potent methodological development that could be used to stimulate global health research, because it greatly simplifies research collaboration. Communication can be established, discussions continued with the aid of (at present) somewhat rudimentary videophone images, and documents worked on cooperatively. Indeed, the development of the technology of computer supported cooperative working (CSCW) on tasks, including the preparation of research reports and papers, is now well advanced.

Nevertheless, available knowledge is sometimes not used, even when its existence is known; why is this? It may be partly a matter of perceptions: perhaps economic (e.g., estimated cost may be too great; judgments about cost in relation to benefit may have been made by inappropriate authorities), perhaps anticipated problems of implementation, including any necessary modifications for local circumstances or perhaps a matter of lack of motivation due to an absence of prior experience of inward transfer of knowledge, technology or know-how, or a reluctance to use ideas from elsewhere.

Within WHO itself, the need to access available knowledge takes a different form. First, there is a wealth of knowledge and experience that has been gained by its professional staff members and external advisors in the course of, for instance, missions to various countries. This often includes valuable insights into country circumstances, economic situation, sociocultural factors and other local details that are not normally part of a formal report. This indicates the need for a specific project, having two main targets:

1. to provide easy access in-house about what the organization "knows", encapsulated in summarized formal reports, extended to capture informal facts, perceptions and judgments obtained by professional staff and external experts about the situation in a country, or about aspects of whatever topic their report concerns and,
2. to set in train a regular in-house practice of providing material for the purpose.

It would be hoped that, through making the stored material available on an intranet, it could and would be readily and regularly accessed by staff within the organization,

---

[1] For details of the *Research policy agenda for science and technology to support global health and development*, see ref. 19. The full text of the *Research policy agenda* is available online at http://whqlibdoc.who.int/hq/1998/WHO_RPS_ACHR_98.1.pdf.

especially if it is made easy for staff to identify documents that are particularly relevant and important to them. It could also improve the opportunities for staff members to see the wider implications of their work for other parts of the organization, and vice versa. The effect of this project would be to implement the first steps towards setting up a "collective memory" and a "collective intelligence" for WHO.

To ensure that this process can become "second nature" within the organization, it is regarded as vital to make full use of the spoken word in capturing this information, so that easy informality can be maintained. This would have the effect of making it easier to express the understanding and insights the experts have been able to gain, and for the nuances of meaning to be captured effectively. At a later stage, the stored information should be structured into a "knowledge base". By searching the documents within which specific topics appear, the stored information can be further explored and enhanced with the aid of "knowledge based" software to yield more general inferences; this would constitute a gain in "knowledge", derived from the available information.

Methods for intersectoral research

Health status depends not only on biological aspects, but on a broader range of other factors that clearly influence health, such as nutrition or the impact of the physical environment. Certain of these factors have been the subject of research but undoubtedly require more attention than they have been given hitherto. But other possible factors affecting health remain very largely unclarified; it might be said that those of specifically socioeconomic origin constitute largely uncharted territory for scientific investigation. Research in this area is regarded as both timely and important, but the techniques for investigation are limited.

Relevant research questions can readily be defined, for example: how the social environment affects health (including the effect of domestic or local violence, civil disturbance and wars, "borders" health) social aspects of urbanization, the influence of the economic environment, unemployment and economic migration.

In order to study such matters, methodologies for identifying and studying interactions between health and activity in other sectors must be developed. One fundamental requirement is a method by which to measure or otherwise evaluate variables in non-health sectors that could be relevant, and correspondingly in the health sector. This requires first, the identification of variables in non-health sectors that can be used as indicators of any suspected health effect and second, the identification of variables in the health sector that reflect this influence. However, many of these variables cannot be expressed numerically. One can envisage, for instance, that a combination of circumstances in a community's socioeconomic situation might constitute the non-health sector "variable"; such circumstances could only be expressed as linked statements of fact. The health sector "variable" under examination might concern, for example, psychiatric illness. If the incidence was in question, the variable would be described numerically; but if the interest was in the nature and related circumstances of the risk of psychiatric illness, numerical measures would not necessarily apply. Methods for analytical, rather than subjective, study of such possible relationship are needed. Research into "knowledge-based" techniques may meet this requirement. Thus, "knowledge" considerations apply to economic and socioeconomic influences on health. Many elaborate econometric models purport to describe the economic system in a country. Their inadequacy in the context of how the economy, or indeed, any non-health sector affects health lies partly in their inability to handle important information that exists only in the form of semantic "knowledge". For instance, motivations derived from prior experience affect how individuals, families and communities use their resources. This could easily be expressed as a verbalized descriptive statement, but not directly as the mathematical expression that econometric models demand. In the study of what factors affect the motivation of people to seek and accept health care, non-health influences would seem to be crucial. These are difficult to study, yet expert observation and inference, organized within various "knowledge-based" techniques, could constitute a useful support to research on such matters.

More generally, inter-sectoral research also will require means to handle non-quantitative information. The basis for inter-relating qualitative and quantitative data is well-founded in human psychology and other social sciences, but only in that restricted context. To meet the needs of global health research, qualitative data could, in principle, be better handled with the aid of technical procedures under the name of "fuzzy measures and fuzzy logic" although health research applications are limited as yet (an interesting early example was the use of fuzzy variables in questionnaires designed to study the relation between social stresses, psychological factors and the incidence of coronary heart disease.) But within intersectoral studies, much relevant information comes in the form of "knowledge" rather than data, so the first step in developing general methodologies for intersectoral research is to provide "knowledge-based" techniques. More experience is needed in applying fuzzy variables and approximate reasoning in global health research.

Knowledge-based techniques depend on three elements: a scheme for provision of the basic information gained by experts, design of the "knowledge map" by which this information is assembled into a usable indicator and the technique to incorporate the indicator- as a variable- into the wider framework of, for instance, an intersectoral model. Each of these elements needs further research and development.

Methods for behavioural research

The influence of behaviour on health is pervasive. "Behaviour" as a concept refers to human behaviours individually, collectively – in groups – and by society generally. It also includes the behaviour of personnel in the health services and in their contacts with one another individually and collectively within the organization, and the way in which the local or overall organization performs both routinely and in the face of large-scale disturbance.

Almost all health problems seem to have an underlying behavioural element. However, identifying important factors affecting health and studying the mechanisms objectively will again require major methodological developments. These will support and extend, if not replace (to some extent) psychological and sociological techniques. It is envisaged that the most important techniques will be based on cognitive science, drawing upon computational logic, guided by *inter alia* anthropological expertise.

Understanding the mechanisms means, to take one aspect of peer group pressure as an example, to clarify how the education and psychological 'set' of an individual renders that individual more or less susceptible to health damaging behaviour patterns that are standard within a group. Insight of this type would be intended, not to provide a basis for designing "behaviour modifiers", but rather to see how motivations develop – with a view to perhaps "motivation modifiers" having potential for improving health.

While quantitative methods are well established in individual psychology and, to an extent, in social psychology as well, these do not fully illuminate the pathways by which behavioural imperatives affect health. On the other hand, there is a multiplicity of potentially relevant factors, particularly in the social or household context, that can again be perceived by experts, although their complexity and number frustrate the unaided attempt to draw systematic conclusions. Expert perceptions can, however, readily be expressed as natural language statements; again the task is to develop techniques to handle extensive information of this kind in an objective way that will lead systematically to valid inferences.

Entire systems also have their "behavioural" characteristics. A recent study of the introduction of computerization into a network of social data-gathering centres in an industrializing country found an extremely high reporting rate of equipment failure. It emerged that, typically, the equipment had not failed; introducing computers into an organizational structure had not considered the social characteristics of the system. Within organizations, behaviour patterns in respect of the way people interact in carrying out their work appear substantially to affect the efficiency of the organization.

Even a virtual research centre formed by the interactive collaboration of several laboratories will develop its own behavioural characteristics. And – a more immediate example – understanding the consequences of introducing new technology into a health system means understanding and taking account of "behavioural characteristics" of the system.

In brief, it is now believed that within organizations, behaviour patterns in respect of the way people interact in carrying out their work appear substantially to affect the efficiency of the organization. Formal methodologies for such studies are not well-known, it they exist at all. Developing and applying appropriate methods to develop "behavioural" methods of health care delivery systems would help design more effective organizations. Such approaches could add an extra dimension to the analysis or design of health care systems at both small and large scales.

"Knowledge-based" assessment of health

Valid observations about health aspects of a community, for instance, made by expert observers, and justifiable insights, would constitute real "knowledge", even if this knowledge did not take the form of numbers. But it would be vital that these inputs be subjected to tests of consistency, and be handled objectively and systematically. Recent technological innovations and developments make it possible to make effective systematic use of verbalized "knowledge" expressed in the form of natural language. It is also possible to employ techniques that, in effect, allow the logical implications of such expert insights to be explored and understood. The use of such "knowledge-based" technologies and "knowledge maps" in the health field may offer the kind of development that is now needed.

Two aspects are required: "fuzzy measures and fuzzy logic" and "computational logic". Fuzzy measures are a natural consequence of using "natural language" to express "knowledge". But "fuzzy" does not mean "sloppy". Rather, it provides a systematic way of handling the complexity of the system with which we need to deal, by allowing "uncertainty" in our descriptions and in our inferences. Computational logic is a means of using logic as a computer language, to handle the "meaning" of verbalized "statements" and to draw logical inferences from these statements. Put briefly, in the present context it is hoped to apply the methodology of computational logic to derive inferences and implications from the observations and insights of expert observers, expressed in "natural language" and using "fuzzy measures" and "fuzzy logic".

Specifically, there is a fundamental need for new and better health status indicators and for indicators to aid research on multi-sectoral interactions with health. The design of a class of "knowledge-based" indicators is therefore an important research target. A "top down" design strategy (one of the approaches) starts with the high level indicator itself (for example, "community health status of the aged') and, by cognitive analysis, decomposes this "concept" into its constituent elements, each of which is analysed in turn, and so on until elements are reached that can be measured or observed. Such basic elements can be illustrated by, for instance, information about typical household arrangements for the aged, community support, physical capability, mental capability, extent of dependence, contribution to the work of the household, health history, prior occupational disabilities, endemic diseases in the community and so on.

Then the process is inverted, and the relations between the various fundamental elements – expressed as semantic statement of "knowledge" or other forms of relation – is used to infer the next higher level element, and so on. The totality of the linkages and the "knowledge" expressing how elements are related constitutes a "knowledge map" of the indicator. The "knowledge map" shows how the "health status" of the aged in the community is "assembled" from the observation of basic facts, in light of other expert insights about relationships. Accordingly, it would also indicate how these basic "determinants" act, and through which pathways, to lead to the picture of "health status" as described.

Understanding the nature of the "health status" indicator resulting from the "knowledge map" requires consideration of the dimensionality of the "high level inferences" generated by the "knowledge map". One approach is to regard the health status indicator as having both positive and negative elements. Aggregated measures of health deficits demonstrated by the "knowledge map" can be compiled into a "severity" element. These elements have different implications, would be used differently and for different purposes, and should therefore be treated as constituting two different "dimensions" in the indicator. The dimensionality would also be increased if it is necessary to take account of consequences that only occur in certain specific circumstances. These are due to "latent" factors and pathways that are only activated in certain circumstances (for instance, the risk of malaria spreading in an afforested region may be zero, even if the insect vector is already present, until non-indigenous workers, who happen to harbour and serve as a "pool" of the disease, enter the region. Again, if a given disease is successfully eliminated from a region by appropriate interventions, it may uncover another disease which is simultaneously present but masked by the first. The second is, in this sense, "latent".)

Similar research developments are needed for the representation of other sectoral variables, for intersectoral studies, leading on the development of methods to model the intersectoral interactions with health using "knowledge-based" indicators.

Health data interpretation

Some health-related data are time-varying (e.g. seasonal outbreaks), some vary spatially (e.g. cases of radiation sickness; breeding sites of insect vectors), some are both (e.g. the spread of a communicable disease). Some data take the form of "point events" occurrences (e.g., cases of disease on a day to day basis, locations of cases within a city, locations of hospitals or health centres). Remote sensing and geographical information systems (GIS) provide the opportunity to link maps with other ground data so that, for instance, the location of new health centres and hospitals can take account of the spatial density and scatter of the populations concerned, the road or river network and any transport facilities serving the area for access.

This type of data can become the basis for useful research. With sufficient reliable data about the spatial location of dwellings, schools, markets and also about the occurrence rate and location of cases of a communicable disease, it is feasible to determine the "operational" – as distinct from the biological – mechanisms for the transmission of the disease, the evolution of its case occurrences and its spatial spread and translation. Pattern analysis is a tool in such studies, which have been carried out with, for instance, variola minor and measles epidemics, and feral rabies epizootics. Given possible outbreaks of communicable diseases for which neither vaccine nor antimicrobials are yet available, this kind of information could be used to plan geographical and community control procedures; it could also throw light on the "operational" characteristics of the spread of communicable disease.

The characteristics of insect vector movement can be tracked in some cases by satellite remote sensing, but in other cases and on a smaller scale, ground radar with supplementary assistance is needed. There are significant opportunities for research with such technology in studying both the role of particular vectors in spreading disease and the behavioural characteristics of the vectors.

Pattern analysis is another methodology which has been developed in the context of several epidemiological problems. It highlights and attempts to explain the underlying systematic patterns, reflecting biological mechanisms that are not often visible in individual or collective records. Various methods have been innovated in the study of weanling diarrhoeal disease, the growth patterns of young infants, the spatio-temporal incidence of fetal abnormalities, the characteristics of blood pressure fluctuations in man and the effect of workload stress (and even of space flight) on physiological mechanisms. The methods rely on being able to recognize various kinds of features in the records. They allow the recognition of common systematic components underlying seemingly intractable variability and generally offer a useful basis for generating hypotheses that can be followed up by scientific investigation. There is scope for much more development of this approach.

Modelling and simulation

Modelling means creating a representation of the structure and function of some real world system; while simulation means using it to determine how the real world system would behave in a given situation. Success requires accuracy and adequate completeness in describing the system. However, a dominant feature of many global health problems is the complexity of the factors involved, of the pathways and systems by which they affect health and the consequential interactions with other, non-health, sectors.

Modelling and simulation research that aims to make a lasting contribution to reducing global health problems needs methodologies to assess health status, to assess the relevant factors affecting health, to describe potentially interacting variables outside the health sector and to tackle "complexity". Much of the data and other information needed are not readily available. Many of the factors and variables may not be measured directly and in any case cannot be expressed quantitatively.

Complex systems do not yield to analysis by the classical approach of disaggregating their component parts. Studying what these parts do in isolation is not useful. Complex systems behave in a way that is determined by how the different components are interconnected and by the interactions between them. So by disregarding the effect of the interactions, one loses any chance of actually understanding how the system works and how it will respond to external interventions. It is not feasible to do experiments on the entire health system to test the effect of different large scale interventions: such an experiment would be too costly, too dangerous and wholly impracticable; nor until very recently, was there any way of studying these sorts of systems as complete structures. The emergence of computer power, especially that based on massively parallel processors, has changed this situation by allowing the possibility of more realistic modelling of such systems. With such models, simulations can be carried out that are equivalent to experimentation in a laboratory.

Examples of models that have been developed in other sectors are: the stock market and city-wide road traffic systems. While of impressively large scale these are, however, essentially of a mathematical kind and need to be developed to handle "knowledge" as well as data to meet at least some of the needs of global research. There is scope for major efforts in modelling and simulation in the global health context. One important task for modelling is to help objectively identify non-health sector influences on health status and the pathways by which they act. If it were possible to "model" these pathways as a "system", strategies for intervening could be identified. Interventions in systems like this cannot necessarily be treated as simple inputs to nodes or as modifications of pathways. A successful intervention would not only generate the intended result, but is likely to have ongoing additional consequences that must be taken into account. It would be difficult to forecast such consequences, and impossible to identify their scope and severity, without a realistic model of the system. Developing such a model would face a special difficulty because it probably could not take on the many varied forms conventionally used in different scientific disciplines. Thus if the model had to use "knowledge-based" indicators – as would seem likely – it would need to comprise at least some aspects that are very different from conventional models, and further research is also needed in this area.

"Behavioural" models of systems, such as health care delivery systems are another important area. Successful developments here would help in designing more effective organizations, adding an extra dimension to the analysis and design processes, at both large and small scales. Even the architectural layout of hospitals has a bearing on how effectively staff interact in carrying out their tasks and, more important, how they react to overloading and to emergencies.

Substantial methodological developments are required in order to provide the means for studying the complex but doubtless important relationships influencing health. This is why early attention to this topic is important.

Priority-setting methodology

As pointed out at the very beginning of the *Research policy agenda*, there can be no simple, single meaning for the concept of "priority". The question is: priority for whom? Every government, people and institution has its own notion of "priority" serving its own purpose, within its sense of mandate, capacity, culture and resources. The scientific community is motivated by the pursuit of intellectual opportunity, but it can be enticed to mobilize and direct its efforts and energies if it knows of the needs and priorities of others. The health needs of humanity are holistic and legion, and so are the research opportunities .The question is whether there are new effective, rational methodologies that can help different parties set priorities for health development research, and perhaps also lead in the direction of a better global consensus. It is clear that the "unfinished health agenda" is enormously complex, and the issues raised encompass very many detailed research problems, not all of which can or should be handled simultaneously with the same degree of effort and prospects of success. How can priorities be set and updated? It is assumed that objective and efficient decision-making is required in this situation. The *Research policy agenda* proposes to put new methodologies at the service of a continuing dynamic process of priority setting.

Criteria for priority-setting

An acceptable list of criteria for priority setting in health research still needs to be agreed. A few possibilities can be mentioned. One relevant criterion is "the scale and urgency of the need, based on health level assessment, and on an understanding of the fundamental causes of the health problem". Others are "the availability of human and other resources to do the work", and "the likely time scale". Equally important are "the consequences in subsequent years of the possible interventions likely to follow from the research", and "the existence of other options for intervention, outside the health sector". Decision-making that neglected such factors would be potentially hazardous and generally unacceptable.

Some of these criteria are non-numerical: they call for human expert judgment and would be described as "knowledge-based". To take such criteria into account needs "knowledge-based" technology. At the same time, it is necessary to remember that in planning actions, whether of research or of interventions, one's freedom to select appropriate and useful actions is frequently circumscribed by the existence of limitations of many kinds. Acceptability, cultural factors, costs, availability of human resources, practicability and such like, are all "constraints" on action. In judging the impact of criteria therefore, it is necessary to bear in mind the constraints because these may dominate the task.

Constraints and resource allocation

There are at least three ways of using criteria. First, one could imagine a computer simulation of how these various criteria contribute to priorities. This approach may be marginally impracticable at the moment. Second, one could generalize the "constraint" concept. Each individual criterion could be transposed into a form that constitutes a "hard constraint" or a "soft constraint" that would limit decision options. A "hard" constraint is one that must not be breached; cultural factors sometimes constitute "hard" constraints. "Soft" constraints are those which are not absolutely forbidden but which are increasingly undesirable as they are increasingly breached. An example is "a short time scale of the research"; the longer the time-scale, the less acceptable on these grounds. Constraints may be expressed in quantitative terms (e.g. the cost limit is USD 20 million), or in the form of specific statements (e.g. the necessary research staff should not exceed number N1 virologists, N2 biochemists, N3 molecular pharmacologists, N4 epidemiologists or X as the case may be). Some constraints need to be expressed in so-called "fuzzy measures". "Likely solutions must be implemented easily" is one example; "the likelihood of success should be fair, good or very good", is another. Other constraints arise in the context of resource allocation because of limitations to implementation. These examples make clear that different research problems would experience different constraints, or at least differently categorized constraints.

Constraint logic programming is a "knowledge-based" technology that is used as further development of logic programming. The strategy of constraint logic programming is to search automatically through many solutions, using the existence and the nature of the constraints to discard those classes of solutions that are unacceptable, and ranking those that are influenced by soft constraints (solutions, in this context, are acceptable options for the distribution of priorities). Part of the skill of the technology of constraint programming is to analyse and use the logical structure of the constraints automatically to make the task of identifying unacceptable solutions into a highly efficient process. Some development work would be required before constraint logic programming can be transposed for the needs of global health.

A third research option exists for the resource allocation problem. This is to construct a special kind of model – a "knowledge map" – that assesses the impact of various criteria, taking into account how they combine and interact, and to what effect, then applying each option individually to determine their level of overall "performance". The high level output from this "knowledge map" is not only how each possibility for action "scores" in terms of the individual criteria, but the inferences about how, collectively, they constrain action.

Applications in health situation analysis also exist for the "knowledge map" methodology, focusing on the fact that health status has both a positive and a negative aspect. Health deficits are those components which should be the first to receive attention, although health deficits need to be interpreted in the light of positive health components. A "knowledge map" of health deficits could be built up from the constraints, and handled by logic programming and by constraint logic programming. If it can be achieved, this would allow, *inter alia*, trial experimentation of the effects of intervention strategies. In fact, it would only point to the consequences for health deficits of the interventions proposed; apparently desirable actions would need to be further considered in respect of their impact on the initially positive aspects of health status. So a "map" of the positive health aspects would then be required.

The same kind of approach could perhaps be used for studying intersectoral effects, because the output of the "map" would also "point" to non-health sector linkages. It is suggested that there could be a generic technology, since the "map" concept can be applied to other sectors.

Technologies based on constraint logic programming are now coming into use for industrial purposes where best possible use of resources is vital. It seems appropriate to envisage their use in the global health research arena, where the problems are more far-reaching and the available resources relatively more constrained.

Annex 3
Lord Zuckerman's statement to the 1975 roundtable meeting[1]

"The topic set for this 'Round Table' invites us to consider the processes whereby one defines what kinds of programme of biomedical research should be encouraged at the national level and also internationally through WHO. In his introductory statement at the start of our meetings, Dr Mahler, the Director-General, gave us his views of the objectives and priorities of WHO. He has also provided us with a statement about the research activities which WHO should encourage in the paper that was released on 29 March 1974, under the title *Reflections on WHO's mission*. The matter of the research programme which should be encouraged by WHO also came up this morning in our discussion of paper 12.1. In introduction I need say no more therefore about the framework within which international programmes of research have to be set.

So far as national programmes go, all that needs to be said at this point is that their formulation is the responsibility of the national governments concerned. On the other hand, we at this meeting have stated the view that biomedical programmes of research should also be encouraged regionally. Lest our discussion this afternoon becomes too diffuse, it would therefore be useful if I set up some markers, recognizing, of course, that these could be placed differently by different chairmen.

"My first generalization is that we are concerned only with the encouragement of worthwhile research. Dr. Mahler has reminded us today how much the scientific community suffers in the wider world from the impression that a vast amount of what is designated research is of poor quality, and that some hardly justifies the description, research. My second generalization is that there are certain problems in the biomedical field which can be tackled only internationally – which means tackled under the auspices of the World Health Organization. For example, yesterday we learnt that what we call diabetes may not be a single disease, but a class of geographically distinct disorders. Clearly a matter of this kind can only be investigated with the help of a coordinating body such as WHO. In this respect the Organization is operating in the same way as international meteorological organizations where it is recognized at the start that major problems relating to climatic changes cannot be dealt with on a national basis.

"At the practical level we have to recognize that research projects fall broadly into one or other of two wide categories. The first comprises those projects which can be shown to have social relevance, and which are selected for enquiry because of this characteristic. Projects of this kind can be again divided into two subcategories; the first constitute

---

[1] This statement was delivered at a roundtable meeting in the context of the 17th session of the ACMR in June 1975.

topics which are selected because they accord with the defined social and economic goals of the countries concerned. The second are those projects within a programme of biomedical research which become a matter of popular demand. The way these demands arise is clear enough. Wants are not recognized until the means are available for their satisfaction. For example, if one were to visit some tribe in, say, New Guinea, which had not been exposed to the outside world, we would find that they have no desire for many things which we, in the kind of civilization in which we live, regard as essential. But once a 'want' is recognized, it becomes a 'need', and soon a need becomes a social demand. From that moment on demands become entitlements, rights which it is assumed everyone has the freedom to demand from the authorities by whom they are governed.

The second category of biomedical research is made up of those projects which are individually generated. We all know there are only a finite number of fields of research interest which are being pursued in the laboratories of the world at any given moment. The research activities of today, the results of which are published widely in scientific journals, are thus essentially a continuation of those of yesterday, in the same way as the present is always an adaptation of the past, and in the same way as the present will project itself into the future.

"But equally, we have to remember that the future is always at the mercy of capricious genius. A future Lederberg, a future Monod are not necessary conditions for the further progress of society. But once genius has declared itself, once it has opened up some new field of intellectual interest, it inevitably qualifies the actions of others, and helps determine the lines of future progress.

"Whether we are dealing with programmes of biomedical research which are socially relevant, or those which are what I have called 'individually generated', they are all subject to certain constraints. The first is the fact that resources are always limited, and that it is consequently necessary for agreement to be reached about the priorities of the various projects which might fit into another category. The second is that the room for manoeuvre open to those responsible for the deployment of research resources is always limited because of previous commitments. The third is that when a new line of research opened up, it frequently happens that older problems become forgotten. Fashion starts playing a part and, in the reinforcement of new success, more difficult issues which have not yielded results in spite of burdensome investigation, tend to be overlaid or brushed aside.

"The fourth is that convention is always a barrier to the acceptance of new ideas, and that convention sometimes becomes overt prejudice. It is worth remembering that the laws of thermodynamics were obstructed in their emergence during the nineteenth century for more that 15 years because of the convention; by which I mean because the new idea did not accord with what was then accepted truth.

"The several generalizations which I have enunciated lead me to a general question which we should face in this discussion. It is one which I believe Dr. Mahler referred to earlier in our proceeding – namely whether it is ever possible for the ranking order of projects in a research programme to parallel the ranking order of health needs.

"This question immediately poses the further question of how one sets about defining health needs. Our discussions have shown that there is a considerable lack of knowledge about many of the factors which relate to different diseases. For example, we do not know about the differential incidence of a disease in relation to the socioeconomic status of its victims or to the occupations which they have filled, or to the environmental condition in which they have lived. In my view health needs will never be defined adequately until a powerful effort is made to provide facts of this kind. These can only be elicited by field enquiries of an epidemiological kind, or by what we have been describing as operational research. The information which would be obtained would allow one to make a first shot at settling out health needs in an order of priority.

"We need to remember, however, that this first approximation would only, as it were, be a single frame in a moving film. Health needs will change with the growth of population, and with changes in its age constitution. In third world countries they also change with increasing industrialization and with increasing urbanization. In other words, one needs to maintain a running survey of health needs, recognizing that these may change not only with socioeconomic advance but also because new genius may generate new approaches to old problems, and totally transform the spectrum of disease in the same way as antibiotics did in their day, and cellular and molecular biology may be doing today.

Having devised a list of health needs, their order of priority needs to be arranged not only in terms of their social significance, but also in accordance with the possibilities of dealing with them in the light of prevailing knowledge, and within the constraints set by the limitations of first-class manpower and of the resources which need to be set aside to keep what manpower there is fruitfully engaged.

"Only when this has been done is it possible to look through a second-order approximation of health needs to see what is missing, to decide whether what has been described in our discussions as "undefined areas of concern", might be worth exploring in the light of the research experience of people who might be available. It is at that stage too, that attention should be given to the desirability of considering the secondary and even the tertiary consequences of solutions being found in some of the major problems which will still be left in a priority list of projects of social relevance.

"WHO has an enormous part to play in all this. We are not dealing with a static situation anywhere, but a dynamic one. As the Director-General reminded us in his opening remarks, malaria was all but eradicated, but is now again becoming a scourge in various parts of the world. Time is not on our side. Population is growing. Poverty is growing. Urbanization is bringing about new environmental problems. In some countries there appears to be a beginning of the breakdown of institutional order. In these circumstances it becomes more and more difficult to transfer knowledge which, if applied, would help achieve the objectives of WHO.

"But whatever part WHO plays, we need also to remember that in the final analysis any programme of biomedical research which becomes the policy of a country, is that country's own national responsibility. We have agreed that biomedical research should be carried out regionally in parts of the Third World, but in doing so we have to recognize that while peaks of expertise exist in many of the countries that are concerned, the plains are more extensive, and that they are dry and arid. The world may be moving more and more towards the sharing of a common culture, but we would be deluding ourselves if we supposed that the more sophisticated kinds of health care which the advanced countries enjoy, can be immediately and easily transported to some countries of the Third World. This consideration should also be in the forefront of our minds as we discuss the main issues which concern this Round Table..."

Annex 4
The final report of Prof. T McKeown, 1988[1]

With its emphasis on equity, acceptability, self-determination and social justice, the concept of primary health care reflects admirably the spirit of the "health for all" commitment introduced at Alma-Ata and reaffirmed at Riga. It is, however, a comprehensive approach which includes all the major developments desirable for health under more or less ideal conditions. In the foreseeable future many Third World countries will be unable to afford all of these developments, and it is therefore necessary to assign priority between them according to their effectiveness.

For this purpose there are two sources of enlightenment to which we can turn: the experience of industrial countries during the last two centuries, and the experience of some developing countries which have made rapid progress during the last few decades. Conclusions from these sources are reasonably consistent particularly on the basic observation that the advances in health were due almost entirely to the decline of mortality from infectious diseases.

In developed countries, the infections declined because of (a) increased resistance brought about by improvements in nutrition and later, to a lesser extent, immunization, and (b) reduced exposure, which resulted from hygienic measures (with respect to water, sanitation, food and housing) introduced progressively from the late nineteenth century.

In developing countries the decline in mortality appears to have been predominantly due to better nutrition, for in some countries which in a few decades have attained Western standards of health, there were no substantial advances in other influences. However there were some other developments which contributed powerfully if indirectly to health: education, particularly of women, equity of access to health resources, political and social will to improve health and above all, control of fertility, which safeguarded the advances from the effects of rising numbers.

Given this assessment of the contribution of different influences, developing countries which do not have the resources needed to provide all the services specified under primary health care (and that is the position of nearly all of them) would be well advised to give high priority to research and services in nutrition, immunization and sanitation. And if limited resources prevent the full provision of sanitary services, as they are

---

[1] Professor McKeown was chair of an ACMR subcommittee on health research strategy from 1983 to 1988, the year in which he died. The report of the subcommittee was issued in 1986 but was updated by Prof. McKeown in the weeks before his death. His update is published here for the first time. Please note that the statistics quoted here may have been revised over time as new data and methodology became available.

likely to do, a large advance can be made by increasing resistance to infection. One cannot overestimate the significance of better nutrition in advances in China and Kerala; indeed there were no substantial improvements in water, sanitation and personal care, and immunization coverage was low.

A decision to give priority to nutrition and immunization would point the way to the research needed for advances in health. The problems are largely of an applied nature, currently referred to as health systems research. Although their character varies considerably between regions and countries, their general nature was outlined in this paper in an assessment of the present position of the major influences.

Introduction

When the Report on Health Research Strategy was presented to the ACMR in 1985 it was suggested that it should be kept under review and revised from time to time in the light of experience. There are a number of reasons why a review seems desirable at this time: (a) some developing countries such as China have advanced rapidly in health and it is possible to learn from their experience, (b) in the last few years there have been important developments related to health strategies in the regions, (c) members of the Sub-Committee on health research strategy have participated in examinations of current research activities in several countries in the Eastern Mediterranean Region, and (d) a recent meeting at Riga has reviewed progress during the last 10 years and has extended beyond the year 2000 the commitment to health for all accepted at Alma-Ata.

The present paper, prepared by the former chairman of the Sub-Committee draws on this varied experience, as well as on ideas outlined in a recently published book "The Origins of Human Disease" (McKeown 1988). This book discusses against an historical and international background many of the issues which confront the Sub-Committee, and its conclusions are included as an Annex to this paper. Although these conclusions are concerned with both industrial and Third World countries, the present paper is limited to developing countries, which the participants at the Riga meeting considered should be given special priority.

When we consider how much is known about the causes of disease it seems surprising that improvements in health have not been more rapid. In large areas of the world, health today is no better than it was in developed countries before the eighteenth century: many children die within a few years of birth and a majority are dead before maturity. Moreover, on the basis of present policies it is questionable whether an acceptable minimum standard of health will be achieved everywhere in the foreseeable future. In some countries the difficulties are compounded by extreme poverty, and by the prevalence of tropical diseases which were absent or uncommon in the developed world. However, the rate of progress is most seriously restricted by the failure to identify the main determinants of health, and to establish priorities in health activities in the light of the conclusions.

An inspection of the research programmes of developing countries will show that there are no well-recognized priorities. Indeed some administrators reject the idea of goal-directed research; they believe that the best results are obtained by finding able investigators and giving them freedom. Inevitably the agenda which results from this approach, in its full or modified form, is unpredictable. Subjects for research could equally well be added or removed from the current programmes, since there is no logical basis for their inclusion.

The failure to establish priorities is also evident in health service policies which largely determine the direction, or lack of direction, in research. In general there is a much greater investment in the treatment of disease than in its prevention, but this has resulted from public demands and medical traditions, rather than from assessment of the effectiveness, or even the humanity of different approaches. Health services are normally considered to comprise the care of the sick and the public health services which have developed since the nineteenth century. These include many services concerned with promotion of health and prevention of disease – sanitation, communicable disease control, maternal and child health, school health, industrial hygiene and the like. But they do not include responsibilities related to basic conditions which also profoundly affect health such as agriculture, housing, education, employment and economic policies. Particularly in developing countries, health standards are determined by government policies as a whole rather than by the limited range of services administered by health departments.

The World Health Organization has made a commendable attempt to establish requirements for health by promoting the concept of primary health care. With its emphasis on equity, acceptability, self-determination and social justice this concept reflects admirably the spirit of the "health for all" commitment endorsed at Alma-Ata, but a brief examination will show that it is a comprehensive statement of all the major influences on health, rather than an assessment of priorities between them.

Primary health care: an all-inclusive approach

The content of primary health care was outlined clearly in the Report of the International Conference at Alma-Ata, "Primary health care should include at least: education concerning prevailing health problems and the methods of identifying, preventing and controlling them; promotion of food supply and proper nutrition; an adequate supply of safe water, and basic sanitation; maternal and child health care, including family planning; immunization against the major infectious diseases; prevention and control of locally endemic diseases; appropriate treatment of common diseases and injuries; promotion of mental health; and provision of essential drugs." Moreover this comprehensive agenda was regarded as a statement of basic requirements, to be supplemented according to the economic and social values of each country and its communities. From this statement it is evident that primary health care, so conceived, covers all the major developments needed for health under more or less ideal conditions. It does not attempt to judge the order in which the developments should be promoted where conditions are far from ideal, as they will be in many countries for a long time to come.

The inevitability of deficiencies, and hence the need for priorities is well illustrated by two of the influences that are most critical for health: nutrition and sanitation. A recent report on the world nutrition situation concluded that malnutrition has decreased in

Asia and Central America, has remained stable in South America and has increased in much of Africa. Since the population of the world is expected to double before it stabilizes, and the population of Africa will increase about six times, on the basis of present policies it seems inevitable that serious food deficiencies will continue well into the next century. And the WHO report on sanitary progress during the present decade makes it evident that we are not in sight of the time when clean water and adequate sanitation will be generally available in developing countries, particularly in rural areas.

Priorities in health policies

Let us now consider the services which should be given priority if health is to advance rapidly. There are two sources of information to which we can turn: one is the experience of developed countries during the last two centuries; the other is the experience of some developing countries which have made rapid progress during the last few decades.

Experience of developed countries

In developed countries the improvement in health since the eighteenth century resulted mainly – until 1900 almost wholly – from the decline in mortality from infectious diseases. The direct influences which led to the decline of the infections were as follows:

1. Increased resistance brought about by:
   (a) Improved nutrition. It was responsible for the advance in health in the eighteenth and nineteenth centuries where exposure to infection was increasing because of rapid population growth and defective hygiene.
   (b) Immunization. It accelerated the decline of mortality in the twentieth century, particularly by reducing the pool of infectious people.
2. Reduced exposure to infection, mainly through hygienic measures applied progressively from the late nineteenth century. The important developments were clean water, improved sanitation and, a little later, advances in the handling of food and improvements in housing. To a limited extent exposure was also reduced by treatment.

However there were other influences which contributed powerfully, although indirectly to health: control of fertility came at precisely the time needed to safeguard the advances from the effects of rising numbers; improvements in education more or less coincided with the advance in health; and economic growth provided the resources which led to a rising standard of living, including most significantly improvement in nutrition and hygiene.

If there were no other knowledge to guide us, it would not be unreasonable to apply this experience of industrial countries to the health problems of the Third World. In doing so, however, we would need to recognize certain differences. First, many of the countries are in tropical or sub-tropical areas where additional problems exist. Second, more is known now about the means of control of disease and some measures – particularly immunization – are much more effective than they were at an early stage in industrial countries. Third, for a number of reasons the time available for improvement in health is shorter, measured in decades rather than centuries according to the timetable accepted by the international community in Alma-Ata. And finally, the order of events is unlikely to be the same as in developed countries, where a century and a half of improved nutrition preceded hygienic and other advances, and the decline of the birth rate occurred at precisely the time needed to limit population growth.

Experience of developing countries

Fortunately additional evidence is now available from a number of Third World countries which have advanced rapidly in health: China, Costa Rica, Cuba, India (Kerala State), Jamaica, Sri Lanka, Thailand and a few others. The conclusions which follow are based on books, papers and case studies which have examined this experience. Two reports have been particularly valuable: in 1984 WHO published case studies from five countries which described linkages between government departments and attempted to assess the relative importance of the influences which contributed to health; and in 1985 another conference sponsored by the Rockefeller Foundation examined data from several countries and drew attention to the need for further research to clarify the effects of different influences.

On what may be regarded as the most basic observation and the starting point for further investigation, the experience of the countries which have recently advanced is consistent with the conclusion based on industrial countries: the improvement in health was almost entirely due to a reduction of deaths from infectious diseases. To assess priorities in health policies in the Third World the chief requirement is therefore to come to a conclusion about the reasons for the decline of the infections. Again, it will be important to distinguish between direct and indirect influences, and it will be convenient to examine the direct influence under the same headings as in developed countries:

1. *Increased resistance to infection*. All of the countries which advanced rapidly achieved a substantial improvement in nutrition which led to increased resistance. Indeed in some countries this was the only important direct influence. It is perhaps surprising that immunization appears to have contributed relatively little to the advances, not of course because it was ineffective, but because the reduction in mortality occurred in a period when vaccine coverage was still low.

2. *Reduced exposure*. Improvements in water supply and sanitation were important influences in industrial countries but they do not seem to have been very significant in the Third World countries which have advanced. For example, the coverage of the population by provision of clean water and safe sanitary measures was low in China, Kerala and Sri Lanka – lower indeed than in many other developing countries – although their death rates were well below average levels. It is also clear that treatment of established diseases contributed little to the reduction of exposure, for in several countries there was little improvement in personal care services.

As in developed countries there are a number of important indirect influences to be considered. In spite of large differences in culture, religion and economic and social conditions, the countries that have advanced all achieved a considerable degree of control of fertility. The limitation of numbers and associated birth spacing undoubtedly contributed largely, if indirectly, to the reduction in mortality, particularly in infancy and childhood. Education was also important: there were notable advances in all the countries, in both primary and secondary education, particularly in the education of women. Although economic development is an important indirect determinant of health, prosperity as indicated by the gross national product or per capita income is not always essential, since the distribution of wealth and the use of resources may be as significant as their creation. Among the countries that have advanced rapidly, China, Sri Lanka and Kerala State are poor as judged by per capita income, and some others are in the mid-range for developing countries. By contrast there are countries with a high per capita income which have shown little improvement. Equity of access to the determinants of health was an important feature in all the countries that have advanced, as was the political and social will to bring about improvements in health. In some countries this will originated from the people themselves, and was largely the result of education which led to awareness of basic human rights. In other countries, and notably in China and Cuba, the political will is centrally directed on behalf of the people.

Although the conclusions from developing countries that have advanced in health are incomplete, they are on the whole consistent with those drawn from experience in the developed world. They suggest that in a Third World country which seeks to progress rapidly, an essential requirement, and in a sense the starting point, is the political and social will to bring about improvement. The initiative may come from the government, as in China, or from the people, as in Kerala, where they have become aware of the possibility of a better and healthier life. This awareness is determined largely by the general level of education, both primary and secondary, and particularly by the education of women. The countries also need to achieve some equality of access to the resources that determine health. Economic development is of course desirable, and in the long term essential, for sustained improvement. Nevertheless some poor countries have reached higher standards of health than others that are wealthier (or more accurately, less poor), by their determination to advance and their acceptance of more even distribution of resources as the necessary means.

But it is important to recognize that although education, equity, economic development and the like are all important, their effects on health are indirect. The direct influences which lead to the rapid decline of infections are (a) increase of resistance from better nutrition and immunization, and (b) reduced exposure mainly through hygienic measures. All have contributed largely in developed countries, but to this point in time the predominant influence in the Third World was improved nutrition.

It follows that developing countries which do not have the resources needed to provide all the services specified under primary health care – and that is the position in which almost all are placed – would be well advised to give high priority in research and services to nutrition, immunization and hygiene. And if the resources available limit full development of sanitary services in the foreseeable future (as they are likely to do), a very large advance can be achieved by increasing resistance to infection. It is hardly possible to overestimate the significance of the observation that in China and Kerala, which in a few decades have reached Western standards of health, the advance was due almost entirely to better nutrition; there were no substantial improvements in water, sanitation and personal care services, and immunization coverage was low.

The present position of the major influences on health in developing countries

To anyone who has travelled extensively in the rural areas of the Third World, the common causes of ill-health may seem self evident. Niamey children are visibly malnourished; sanitary conditions are primitive, drinking-water is unclean, the food displayed in open markets is contaminated; and the number of people competing for the means of life is clearly excessive. Our conclusions concerning the determinants of health can be epitomized by the simple statement that the most elementary requirements are that people must have enough to eat and they must not be poisoned. The frequency and causes of food deficiencies and hygienic hazards have been examined in numerous reports by the World Bank, the World Health Organization and the United Nations, and the conclusions that have been drawn will be summarized in relation to the critical influences; food, immunization, drinking-water, sanitation and control of numbers.

Food

A World Bank study of the relation between poverty and hunger quoted an edict by the Emperor Wen in 113 BC: "Why is the food of the people so scarce? Where does the blame lie?" The deficiency is ever more remarkable today, because in many countries and in the world as a whole food supplies are believed to be adequate. The World Bank Study concluded: "The often predicted Malthusian nightmare of population outstripping food production has never materialized. Instead the world faces a narrower problem; many people do not have enough to eat despite there being food enough for all. This is not a failure of food production, still less of agricultural technology. It is a failure to provide all people with the opportunity to secure enough food – something that is very hard to do in low-income countries." Although one would question the statement that population growth has never outstripped food production, it is an accurate assessment of the position in many countries today.

In relation to health, our interest is in the frequency of malnutrition and the reasons for its occurrence when food supplies are adequate. The World Bank Study used two criteria to assess the position in 1970 and 1980.

> "Between 340 million and 730 million people in the developing countries did not have enough income to obtain enough energy from their diet in 1980. The estimate of 340 million is based on a minimum calorie standard that would prevent serious health risks and stunted growth of children. If the standard is increased to levels that allow an active working life, however, the estimate rises to 730 million. About two-thirds of the undernourished live in South Asia and a fifth in sub-Saharan Africa. In all, four-fifths of the undernourished live in countries with very low average incomes."

The recent First Report on the World Nutrition Situation (1987) made an appraisal of trends in nutritional indicators from 1960 until the most recent year available, usually

1985. The report concluded that although nutrition has improved over the last 25 years in most parts of the world, in sub-Saharan Africa there has been declining food availability and increased malnutrition, and in South America there has been no significant improvement. Improvements in living conditions recorded during the 1970s have slowed or halted with the severe economic recession of the early l980s, and this is affecting child nutrition.

In light of our conclusion concerning the critical role of nutrition, the data for China in this report are of particular interest. Over the past 25 years, China's per capita food production increased 75% and its population by around 60%; dietary energy supply increased from less than 1800 kcals/capita/day in 1961/1963 to 2560 in 1983/1985. There were corresponding increases in birth weights and child growth rates, and infant mortality fell from 200 (per 1000 live births) before 1949 to about 40 in 1980, and to 35 in 1982. As already noted, apart from the improvement in nutrition there were no other major changes which could account for the reduction in mortality.

The increased food production during the last 35 years has resulted mainly from technological advances, the use of chemical fertilizers and pesticides, increases in the amount of irrigated land and the introduction of high yielding disease resistant seeds. As a result of these advances, grain production more than kept pace with the growth of populations, both in the world at large and in developing countries considered as a whole. However, for a number of reasons the practice of equating food resources with the number of people gives a misleading picture of the effects on nutrition.

First, even by the simple test which relates resources to population, many countries do not have enough food. In 1977-1980, one-third of the population of the Third World lived in countries where supplies – output, stocks and imports – were insufficient to provide everyone with an adequate diet, even if distributed according to need. The position is particularly serious in Africa, but there are also countries in Latin America and South Asia where output per head has fallen.

A second reason for concern is that several countries, which by the simple test relating resources to numbers may be said to have enough food, have only a small margin, and are ill-equipped to meet transitory deficiencies. These arise for a number of reasons: unstable world prices, variation in domestic production, variation in household purchasing power and famine. Famine is the most severe source of transitory deficiency and it may have several different causes. Investigation of some serious famines has shown that a reduction in the food available is not always the primary reason, and attention is increasingly focused on other causes, particularly loss of real income.

A third reason, and the most common, for the inadequacy of food to population arithmetic is that the food available is very inadequately distributed, both between countries and between different areas and population groups in the same country. India, for example, has an overall food surplus which more than kept pace with the phenomenal increase of population; yet for several years there has been acute famine in the north among the eight million people who live in the arid region of Rajasthan.

Against this background it is evident that malnutrition and its sinister effects on health are common in developing countries, and result mainly from international and national policies which prejudice food production and distribution. The international community can contribute in many ways – with resources, with advice and not least by refraining from encouraging or requiring Third World countries to absorb food surpluses (the grain and butter mountains) or to adopt agricultural and economic policies which contribute to their poverty. However, the causes of food insecurity and the resultant ill-health are determined largely by national policies. The chief requirements are (a) to ensure an adequate food supply through policies which promote domestic production (by shifting resources from industry to agriculture, from large to small farms, from capital-intensive to labour-intensive activities) and (b) to give people at risk of food insecurity the opportunity to earn an adequate income. The problem of food deficiency is determined essentially by poverty.

Immunization

Our assessment of priorities in health research and service policies was based on the experience of developed countries and of the handful of developing countries which have recently advanced. Relying on this evidence from the past we are likely to underestimate the contribution that immunization can make to the control of infectious diseases in the future. This risk arises because mortality from many infections had declined to quite a low level mainly because of other influences – nutrition and hygiene in industrial countries and nutrition in the Third World – before effective immunization was widely applied. It is therefore essential to reassess the contribution which may be expected from immunization in the light of current knowledge of its potential. This contribution has been assessed by Professor Danielsson and I cannot do better than quote from his paper on Biomedical Research and its Impact on Health Care.

> "Infectious diseases, be they of bacterial, parasitic or viral origin, can be considered in a worldwide perspective to be the most important group of diseases to combat. At the present state of knowledge this combat will likely be more successful in a 10-15-year perspective than that directed at many other diseases. The major factors behind this supposition are the advances in molecular biology and immunology. The knowledge about the chemistry of microorganisms and the mechanisms of their replication offer possibilities to produce vaccines specific for important structures responsible for infectivity of the microorganisms. At the same time, this way of attacking the problems of vaccine production decreases or eliminates unwanted side-effects of vaccines. Recombinant DNA technology has provided an instrument to prepare immunogenic material at reasonable cost. A particular advantage with this technology is that deletion mutants which lack certain virulent genes can be prepared. These mutants will be antigenic but will be safer than vaccines prepared according to procedures currently used. Another possibility for vaccine production involves utilization of subunits or components of microorganisms. Such vaccines will contain parts that are antigenic but lack components that may cause infections or other unwanted side-effects. Still another approach is to prepare vaccines containing crucial, antigenic peptides. The possibilities of this procedure are difficult to assess at present. There is a problem of protein conformation, i.e. that these peptides must resemble in a three-dimensional way the structure of the whole protein in the membrane of the microorganism.

> "Vaccines may also be constructed as anti-antibodies which act as antigens and elicit immune response. There is already experience from experimental systems that such anti-idiotypic

vaccines are effective in viral diseases such as hepatitis, influenza and poliomyelitis, and in parasitic diseases such as trypanosomiasis.

"In recent years, increased attention has been directed towards the use of viral vectors as a means of carrying antigens. The idea is that the live virus, e.g., vaccinia, will express a foreign gene inserted into its DNA when it is applied to an animal. This will subsequently lead to an immune response to the product of the foreign gene. Immune response has been shown in animals with vaccinia as a vector for immunization against, for instance, hepatitis B and herpes simplex. A drawback is that there may still be a high level of immunity to the vaccinia virus in the population. The principle can, however, be applied with other viruses as vectors, e.g., adenovirus and herpes virus.

"When parasites are considered, e.g., malaria, it can be assumed that vaccines will contain proteins from different stages of the evolution of the parasite. By such a design it will be possible to attack the parasite at different stages of its life cycle. However, it should be borne in mind that it is an enormous task to delineate which structures constitute the major antigens. Research dealing with malaria has progressed the farthest. So far, interest has focused on the sporozoite stage of the malaria parasite. Two vaccines consisting of the linear epitopes of the circumsporozoite protein have been produced and are being tested clinically. The first vaccine is a synthetic peptide coupled with tetanus toxoid, which serves as a carrier. The second vaccine, which has been produced by recombinant DNA technology, consists of 32 four-amino-acid repeat units from P. falciparum circumsporozoite protein and a tail, 32 amino acids long, encoded by the vector. The trials indicate some success with these vaccines. Already, a second generation of vaccines is in preparation. In this case, the work involves defining epitopes of the malaria parasite that stimulate T-cells and thereby result in induction of cellular immunity. The rationale of this work is that efficient protective immunity can only be obtained when both arms – humoral and cell-mediated – of the immune system have been activated. To underline the importance of this, it might be mentioned that sporozoite-infected hepatocytes are only susceptible to cell-mediated immunity and not to antibodies.

"A problem with vaccines that is not yet satisfactorily solved at present is that of adjuvant. To make the vaccines optimally effective, adjuvants are needed. It can he assumed that research on the regulation of the immune system will provide knowledge about suitable and effective compounds that stimulate the immune system.

"In discussing vaccine production the role of the use of monoclonal antibodies should not be overlooked. Monoclonal antibodies constitute an invaluable instrument to define antigens relevant for induction of protective immunity or mediation of pathological response. They can be employed in purification of antigens to be used as vaccines.

"Even if the advancement in techniques for vaccine production, as outlined above, is remarkable, there are many problems that await their final solution. This is best exemplified by the case of AIDS. Present knowledge about the molecular biology and virology of the HIV viruses is substantial. Yet, there is no vaccine available and it may take many years before one becomes available. The unique pathogenicity and variability of HIV virus have raised new challenges in vaccine design, testing and evaluation. In HIV, the external portion of the envelope glycoprotein is a major target for both antibody-mediated neutralization and cytotoxic immunity and this glycoprotein has been considered a good candidate for an AIDS vaccine. Various ways have been used to produce a pure antigen. The native glycoprotein has been isolated from HIV-infected human cell lines and a recombinant form as well as the whole envelope gene product has been expressed in mammalian cell systems. Furthermore, a 180 amino acid part of the glycoprotein and a synthetic peptide have been produced. In other experiments, a peptide derived from a protein located immediately underneath the viral envelope has been synthesized to produce a possible subunit vaccine. The rationale of this approach is that this protein is highly conserved among HIV variants in contrast to the envelope protein. Experiments have also been performed in which the HIV viral envelope has been inserted into live virus vectors. Finally, attempts have been made to use anti-idiotypic antibodies to either the HIV envelope or its natural receptor on lymphocytes. In summary, a number of techniques have been tried in attempts to prepare a vaccine against AIDS and several trials have been carried out or are being carried out in monkeys and humans to test preparations for their efficacy as vaccines. So far, the results are not too encouraging."

Overall, the prospects to combat infectious diseases in the coming decade seem good and can be mostly attributed to breakthroughs in biomedical research like recombinant DNA technology and monoclonal antibodies. It should be added that basic biomedical research also will provide better instruments for vector control. Suffice it to mention elucidation of the chemical structures of many sex attractants in insects.

Although vaccination coverage was low in most of the developing countries that have advanced, immunization of the world's children is now increasing quite rapidly. In 1987, 50% were protected against tuberculosis, diphtheria, whooping-cough, tetanus, poliomyelitis and measles; ten years earlier the proportion was 5%. Unfortunately, the level of coverage is lowest in developing countries for two diseases which cause many deaths, measles and neonatal tetanus. Nevertheless, recent appraisal suggests that prospects for the future are quite bright: by the year 2000 poliomyelitis should be eradicated, deaths from neonatal tetanus should disappear, and mortality from measles should be reduced by 95%.

If we are to rely largely on improvements in nutrition and immunization for rapid advances in health in the Third World – and this is the conclusion which emerges from our assessment of the major influences – it is important to consider the relationship between the two. WHO emphasizes that it is essential to vaccinate children even if they are malnourished or suffer from minor illnesses. But although the presence of malnutrition does not make it undesirable to immunize, it is also true that the availability of immunization does not make it unnecessary to prevent malnutrition. It would be an unsatisfactory policy to protect children from some diseases by vaccination, only to have them die from malnutrition or other diseases (such as pneumonia or diarrhoea) related to malnutrition. The correct approach is surely to provide both services, and in most countries, perhaps in all, this can be done if they are given the priority that their contributions seem to justify.

Drinking-water and sanitation

We must now consider one of the most common natural hazards, the pathogens that cause the diarrhoeal diseases which kill a considerable proportion of all children within a few years of birth. In Latin America in 1978 they were responsible for a quarter of the deaths of children under five years of age, and in 1980 they produced about 4.6 million deaths (under five years) in developing countries. Eighty per cent of the deaths were in children under the age of two.

Because of the seriousness of diarrhoea in children, strenuous efforts are being made to treat the diseases by oral rehydration therapy, and to reduce the frequency and severity of infection by breast-feeding, good nutrition and certain vaccinations. But if health is to improve rapidly it is also necessary to prevent transmission of the pathogens which cause diarrhoea. The measures required are improvements in water supply, in excreta disposal and in domestic and food hygiene. These are the services which led to the rapid decline in deaths from intestinal infections in industrial countries in the late nineteenth and early twentieth centuries.

Attention has been focused internationally on the prevention of diarrhoeal diseases by the United Nations General Assembly which designated 1981-1990 as the International Drinking Water Supply and Sanitation Decade. The measures with which advance is required are:

1. An adequate supply of clean water in or close to people's homes.
2. Hygienic disposal of excreta by ready, and preferably exclusive, access to a hygienic toilet or latrine.
3. Improvements in personal hygiene which ensure that facilities are correctly used and supported by other measures such as hand-washing, hygienic disposal of stools of young children, and improved water storage and food hygiene.

The World Health Organization is monitoring progress during the decade and the most recent report is for the period to the end of 1983. The level of services available in developing countries was summarized as follows:

1. Three urban residents out of four had access to a safe water supply and about 80% of them were served by a house connection,
2. A little over half of urban residents had access to adequate sanitation. Two rural dwellers out of five had access to a safe and adequate water supply. This is regarded as the most significant global achievement in the field of hygiene in recent years.
3. One rural dweller out of seven has access to appropriate sanitation. This is the service where least progress has been made and most needs to be done.

Against this background it is clear that a large increase in the rate of progress will be needed if the targets set for the decade are to be achieved. In the countries that have provided data, in urban areas an additional 186 million residents will have to be provided with water and 200 million with sanitation; in rural areas the corresponding numbers are 643 million for water and 287 million for sanitation. Moreover, these increases are needed, not to provide full coverage of the populations, but to achieve the relatively low targets that have been set for 1990. In the case of rural sanitation, for example, the aim is only to increase coverage to 33% of households, and even this modest advance will probably be beyond the means of some countries.

Countries were asked to give reasons for the limited progress in provision of water and sanitation. The three most important constraints in all regions were lack of funds, insufficient personnel and inadequate operation and maintenance. Their relative importance varied between regions: shortage of funds was the first constraint in Africa and South Asia; in the Eastern Mediterranean it was ranked equally with inadequate water resources; in the Western Pacific it was said to be second to lack of trained staff (skilled artisans and tradesmen). However, all the major constraints are profoundly influenced by the resources available, so that the hazards attributable to inadequate water supplies and sanitation in developing countries are again due to poverty.

Control of numbers

When assessing prospects for health in the Third World, it is important to keep in mind the significance of the timing of the major influences. In industrial countries they became effective in what was, for health and welfare, the ideal sequence. The first and most potent influence on mortality was improvement in nutrition, a consequence of a rising standard of living which preceded hygiene and other measures, in some countries by more than a 100 years. These later measures led to a further reduction of mortality, but their effect on population growth was restricted because they coincided with – indeed in France they were preceded by – a decline of the birth rate brought about by control of fertility. With expansion of food supplies and limitation of population growth an essential requirement was met, a balance between food and numbers which did not provoke Malthusian adjustment through increased mortality. Populations expanded, but at a rate more or less consistent with health needs.

In many developing countries, the time sequence of the major influences is quite different; the application of technological measures has preceded the capacity to provide sufficient food or limit numbers. In Africa, for example, before 1950 the rate of population growth was a little over 1% per year and never exceeded 1.6%; today the average rate is about 3%. The reasons for this increase are not entirely clear, but it appears to have been due largely to the application of biomedical technology. Many of the endemic plagues of Africa have lost their demographic impact. Smallpox has been wiped out; yellow fever is under control in many countries and, when it flares up, it is quickly contained; and malaria can be controlled or limited in its impact. Droughts and famines are not as devastating to human lives as they were in the past. Relief services, although poorly organized, do make a difference in development. All these gains can be increased many-fold with a more extensive application of the already proven intervention technologies. Thus, unlike the historical situation where economic development led the way to and accompanied population increase, in Africa populations are increasing so fast as to frustrate development efforts!

Many estimates have been made of the possible consequences of the present rates of population growth. The most obvious result will be a large increase in numbers of people and it will be greatest in the poorest countries. Projections by the United Nations suggest that the world population, now about 5 billion, will be 6 billion in the year 2000, 8 billion in 2025 and 10 billion before it stabilizes in about 2100.

The rates of increase are very different in different parts of the world. In Europe, North America, Japan and the Soviet Union, fertility has declined rapidly and is now at or near the level needed to maintain stable populations of about the present size. Fertility has also declined in some developing countries in Latin America and East Asia, most notably in China, where there has been a spectacular fall. But elsewhere in the Third

World – Africa, West Asia, South Asia and parts of Latin America – there has been no significant reduction of fertility, and populations are expected to continue to grow at about the present rates. According to medium-term United Nations projections, before stability is achieved the population of 1980 will have increased nearly six times in Africa, about three-and-a-half times in Latin America, and will have doubled in Asia.

Another consequence of present demographic trends is the movement of people, as migrants from one country to another, but even more seriously from the point of view of health and welfare, from rural to urban areas within the same country. In 1983, there were 26 cities with populations over 5 million with a combined population of 252 million. It has been estimated that by the year 2000 there are likely to be 60 such cities with a combined population of 650 million; 45 of them will be in the developed world. Several of the largest cities, such as Mexico City, Sao Paulo and Calcutta will have over 20 million people. Moreover, the migration, formerly confined to capital cities, has begun to affect cities of secondary and even tertiary size, and many are now growing at a much faster pace. The urban migrants have already created formidable problems with respect to food, hygiene, education, housing and health; and it must be remembered that they have moved to the cities, not because they could be assured of employment, but because conditions in rural areas are very bad. "Migrants into towns are at best underemployed and are usually unemployed, creating high crime rates in the shanty towns in which many must live. Often these septic fringes to the towns have vital statistics that are much worse than those of the rural areas."

In view of these conditions it seems remarkable that there should be doubts in some of the poorest countries about the need to restrain population growth. But the control of numbers is an emotive subject which touches on national, religious and racial sensibilities, and there are differences of opinion on whether rapid population growth should be treated as a consequence or cause of underdevelopment. Clearly it is both. Since the nineteenth century it has been evident that birth rates decline as economic conditions improve, and if resources were managed efficiently and distributed equitably between and within nations, the need to restrict numbers probably would not arise, or would not arise yet. But in the world as it exists these requirements will not be met, and limitation of numbers is an essential complement of the measures that need to be taken – particularly sustained economic growth and more equitable availability of wealth. The link between health, numbers and socioeconomic development is widely recognized, and few countries now question the need to lower rates of population growth. Nevertheless, the setting of population targets is still a sensitive and divisive issue, and the control of numbers is not always given the attention in national planning that on health and other grounds it clearly requires.

Annex 5

Recommendations from the World Health Assembly technical discussions, 1990[1]

1. The priorities for action which follow were formulated within the context of several general considerations.

1.1 Variability among countries

It was recognized that there is considerable variability among countries in the capacity to generate and to utilize the results of health related research. This capacity relates to such variables as country size, population, gross national product and the level of industrialization. Consequently, when action at country level is at issue, it may be useful to consider three categories of countries:

a) Countries which have a well-established research infrastructure and career ladder. In such countries, the effort would be to refine and improve. It would not be contingent on significant external support. Such countries might provide examples for those in the other two categories.

b) Those which have made some headway but still require considerable developmental efforts. Countries in this category would probably require external support in attempting to make further progress.

c) Countries with constraints which significantly limit their potential to produce research. In such countries, the focus will probably be on ways of gaining access to and adapting findings from research conducted elsewhere. Under these circumstances, there would be a need to develop at least a minimal capability for evaluation of existing and novel health measures.

1.2 Focus at country level

It was recognized that issues related to health research career structures can be most effectively addressed at country level. Whether a career structure is needed – and if so, how it can be adapted to national priorities, resources and constraints – could be determined through problem-oriented country reviews. The goal is to increase national capabilities to conduct research by adapting the research career structures to national needs. The approach, therefore, will vary as a function of differences among countries as described above.

Effort at regional and global levels in support of country activities will be required. In this respect, many of the priorities for action enumerated below involve a regional or

---

[1] See reference (5).

global component. WHO's activities in this respect should respond directly to country needs.

1.3 Better utilization of existing resources

It was recognized that particularly in times of economic difficulties, ways of using existing resources more effectively are necessary. A number of priorities for action are therefore concerned with methods of increasing national capabilities to better utilize health research as a tool for solving priority health problems. Others address the issue of how existing health research manpower and facilities might be used more efficiently and effectively to generate appropriate research.

2. The priorities for action would include:

2.1 Strengthening national socioeconomic development policies, strategies and plans

(i) Sensitization of decision-makers

The extent to which national level research efforts can be strengthened by the establishment of functional career structures will be determined by the priority governments accord to the role of research as a tool for socio-economic development. Every effort would therefore have to be made to convince national authorities at the highest level of the crucial role of science, technology and research in development. Meetings of the Regional Committees, Regional Advisory Committees on Medical Research, the World Health Assembly provided excellent opportunities for the initiation of such discussions. Of equal importance are the opportunities offered by UN fora to convince national polity planners of the importance of Health Research for National Development.

(ii) Inter-sectoral coordination

National authorities would also have to be convinced of the importance of establishing functional mechanisms for promoting active inter-sectoral coordination between health and health-related Ministries and Departments as well as between Ministries of Health, Faculties of Medicine with special emphasis on their Department of Community Medicine, Research Institutes and the managers of national health care delivery systems. In this respect, the role of National Research Councils and Science Academies as well as national scientists cannot be over-emphasized.

Because of the intimate interrelationship which exists between the establishment of a viable health research programme and the existence of clearly defined research priorities deriving from national health plans and policies and the identification of priorities for research are matters of the greatest importance.

2.2 Strengthening of National Health Research Management

In the group of countries where there is as yet no independent research capability, Ministries of Health could be supported by the creation of a few posts and/or by the provision of technical expertise to assist them to acquire the relevant literature and information already available and to establish practical health information systems to assist them in their planning functions. In other countries attention would have to be paid to ensure that research priorities focus more sharply on the solution of current and more urgent problems and that some research becomes an integral part of programme operation and implementation. This would also help to ensure that these operational programmes and the research itself are made maximally cost-effective and cost-beneficial in terms of their impact and help to convince decision-makers that such research may more than pay for itself. Managers of health services would also have to implement measures to ensure the maximal utilization of the existing resources, derives procedures for the utilization of trained researchers even on a part-time basis, and provide for the more active participation of trained personnel from Departments of Community Medicine and other such training and research institutes in non-governmental sectors. Research managers would also have to assist in the formulation of research manpower development plans which are consonant with the health research plan and ensure that the training is relevant to their future needs. Efforts would have to be directed at making these training programmes "home country"-based to the maximal extent possible, and at exploring and using other training processes.

2.3 Establishment of career structures

The development of career structures must take into account a complex series of factors:

— method of attraction and selection of candidates for a research career;
— remuneration and salary structure of research workers;
— system of promotion;
— work tenure;
— provision of opportunities for part-time workers and of lateral mobility;
— incentive and fringe benefits (special allowances, sabbatical leave, etc.);
— peer evaluation and supervision;
— appropriate working and living conditions;
— availability of adequate funds for research;
— mechanisms for the adequate remuneration of scientists.

Three possible mechanisms could be considered:

— a permanent civil-service-type structure for research workers with its salary scale, channel of promotion, etc;
— recruitment of scientific research staff into the general public service of the country but with a special provision of a research subsidy;
— providing the same conditions of services as university teachers including conditions for recruitment and promotions.

The proposed career structures should make provision for senior scientists to remain in active research should they so desire, rather than have to move to managerial and administrative positions for promotional reasons.

In creating career structures, attention needs to be paid to the problems arising out of long-term tenures. A career ladder where all available positions have been occupied by younger staff members with long-term tenure could well restrict the entry of more senior personnel who have already established their worth.

3. The coordination role of WHO

3.1 Global level

   a) catalytic;
   b) sensitization of government to recognizing basic scientific needs and the identification of health-related research priorities;
   c) support appropriate initiatives at creating and re-enforcing relevant research career structures in developing countries.

3.2 Regional level

   a) To promote inter-regional and intra-regional collaboration in research promotion through joint research projects, seminars and workshops and other forms of regional cooperation including TCDC.
   b) To organize special meetings and workshops to review case studies prepared by countries in the region in order to build some career structures. These meetings will provide opportunities for countries to coordinate their activities in the area of institutional strengthening.
   c) To promote linkages between scientific institutions in the region for the purpose of sharing research management experiences especially in the area of research career structures as well as organization of group training activities and the collaboration between institutions and individual scientists.

3.3 Country level

   a) Focus on national efforts: increase in the capabilities of participating countries to conduct health research by supporting efforts to strengthen their research career structure.
   b) Problem-oriented reviews by national review teams resulting in recommendations for change as necessary.
   c) Sharing of experiences among participating countries and subsequent dissemination to other Member States.

Annex 6
Extract from Research for health: principles, perspectives and strategies, 1993[1]

Research needs and new methodologies

Three issues that arise in the context of health-related research need clarification:

a) Established professional techniques much be applied in order to acquire information about needs, identify technical means and make effective use of those means to meet those needs. Not all of these might be regarded as research in the sense of seeking or extending knowledge and capability, yet their application calls for the allocation, use and evaluation of resources.

b) Methodological innovations or developments may be needed to acquire appropriate information, decide priorities, allocate resources and put research findings into effect.

c) Where new knowledge is required in order to solve existing or emerging problems, goal-specific or strategic research is unavoidable.

Gathering information about health problems, health care facilities and the efficacy and effectiveness of health care delivery is vital for planning the best provision of health care when resources are limited. The use of advanced information technology may be justified in view of the scale and importance of the information sought. Methodological developments may then be needed before the system is designed or the equipment chosen and installed; the failure of some information systems in developing countries has proved to stem from taking insufficient account of cultural and behavioural factors.

The need for new indicators is self-evident in view of all the elements that have a bearing on health. Such elements as quality of life, risks due to environmental hazards and exposure to stress, violence or health-damaging behaviour can be observed and even measured. Their effect on health can rarely be expressed mathematically or modelled conventionally, but is usually expressed in terms of "knowledge", i.e. statements of fact observed or expert belief. Modelling may be possible, but it depends on the use of new forms of representing information, and new methodologies. Similar arguments apply when indicators are required for other health-related or socio-economic variables that cannot be directly observed or measured, and so have to be indicated. Consequently new forms of indicators, and new ways of systems modelling will need to be developed

---

[1] For details of Research for health: principles, perspectives and strategies, see ref. 18. The full text of the document can be accessed online at http://whqlibdoc.who.int/hq/1993/WHO_RPD_ACHR_(HRS)_93.pdf).

in the near future. They will be particularly important when the impact on health of activity in other sectors of the economy has to be established.

Techniques for the utilization of knowledge

Whenever a research solution leads on to an intervention in order to influence the quality or impact of available health care, consequences beyond those immediately targeted will inevitably follow. This should be understood, preferably in advance of the intervention itself. Interventions sometimes lead to very complex consequences: across domains and across sectors. This is the reason for realistic "modelling" of a system: the consequences of the intervention can be tried out on the model.

However the present technology for modelling is wholly inadequate for the kind of socio-economic system that health planners have to handle. It is obvious that quantitative data and relationships are required for econometric-type analysis; when observational and factual 'knowledge' about the system can also be incorporated, a substantial advance in capability will occur. The technology for representing "knowledge" – in the form of textual statements – by computer is well-established and so is the means for making logical inferences using textual knowledge. Research using computational logic will be the key to designing new types of indicators and to modelling and understanding socioeconomic systems; it will extend system modelling from mathematical formulae into the domain of "knowledge-based" systems that are much closer to real life than the models at present available.

Relevance of the economic environment to health

Affordable health care is dictated everywhere by economic factors – at the macro-level through the allocation and distribution of national resources; at the meso-level through the use made of those resources; at the micro-level through the impact of family budgets on health care. National policy, often driven by international forces, dictates the resource allocation for health in the light of national economic needs, but it is recognized – in turn – that the health status of the population may influence the nature and pace of economic development. Limiting the resources made available to the health care delivery system not only increases the problems of managing the health system itself, but also demoralizes the personnel who operate the system.

Consequences of structural adjustment

The impact of national policies on health is a central issue. It is particularly significant where structural socioeconomic adjustment policies have been put into effect, since these have a major social impact, including on health. In fact, their damaging effects on health hit hardest at the household level and on those least able to resist them.

When policies of adjustment take effect, three types of consequence may follow in the health sector: a direct effect on health (e.g. a shift from foodcrops to export products will have a negative impact on nutrition), deterioration of health services because resources no longer flow, lower rewards and incentives for personnel in the health sector leading to a descending cycle of lower morale and, subsequently, lower standards.

Accordingly, much more needs to be known about the effects of adjustment, people's attitudes to those effects, means of ameliorating the consequences for the most needy, and the design of administrative structures to face up to the changed economic scene. For example, what distinguishes countries that have coped successfully with the consequences of adjustment from those that have not? How important are the determinants of organizational behaviour at the managerial level?

It may be possible to identify most of the significant influences on health from outside the health sector, and such information could be used to design integrated policies that target the most effective services to those most in need, by the most appropriate allocation of funds expenditures both within and outside the health sector. External social and cultural factors may be determinants of demand for health care services; for instance, the absences of health services in rural areas may be one factor that tends to drive people to cities. Various models of health care systems are in existence but, whatever the specific system adopted, effective monitoring is needed.

Health and national economic development

In order to achieve targets for meeting health needs in the light of costs, priorities have to be determined. Health needs and circumstances alter dynamically and so do the demands imposed on the health care service. As national circumstances alter, the process must be repeated and must be as dynamic as the system driving it. A taxonomy of needs must therefore be established, and the consequences of intervention in the health sector also need to be classified. This is why modelling, if at all feasible, is important since it provides a means of testing for such consequences and for the effects of intersectoral interaction.

The relative efficiency of different kinds of health sector expenditure in terms of improving health does need to be measured, but the methodology is not available. For example, in the national context, the distribution of resources, functions and activities between public and private sectors or between PHC and hospital care, the influence of user fees and insurance schemes, equity and the protection of the poor – all these call for investigation in both developed and developing countries.

Determinants of health need not only originate in the health sector; there are numerous multisectoral contributions. For instance, economic factors affect health through social provision, housing, availability of suitable food, quality of nutrition and so on; industrialization influences health through the availability and nature of employment, environmental effects, consumption or creation of foreign currency for health- or nutrition-related products and perhaps through the provision of health-related products. Conversely, health affects other sectors. Health is a factor in the physical and mental quality of manpower, in the sickness-absence record in employment, as well as in the consumption of resources that could otherwise be used for economic or social development. Hence the interactions should be investigated, in order to provide a rational basis for forecasting, planning and resource allocation at the national level, within all the sectors, including that of health.

There is a time lag between interventions and disturbances in large-scale economic and societal systems and the consequences that they produce. In this sense, the system is dynamic and hence long-term monitoring and trend assessment are important.

Annex 7
Recommendations from the colloquium on "The impact of scientific advances on future health" (excerpts)[1]

Applied science

Technological advances have led to many new diagnostic and therapeutic possibilities, many of which are costly. Imaging technologies, new materials for internal or external prosthesis, laser technology, biosensors, and silicon chips are examples. Information technology allows effective gathering and utilization of public health information, modern computing technology and the use of computational logic provide new opportunities for systems modelling and for the use of advanced decision support at all levels.

Inequities are easily created by such advances in science and technology. Deciding how and where to allocate resources to the new opportunities may be difficult. Human factors constitute important elements in identifying what health care is acceptable and in designing systems through which health care personnel provide acceptable health care services. Development of technological hardware for developing countries should be directed towards robust, cheap and readily maintained equipment.

Among the basic needs of direct technological concern is the supply of clean water, the provision of sewage disposal, the need for attention to environmental pollution and to industrially-linked disease and disability, methods for early warning of developing health hazards and problems, support devices for the disabled and the elderly, reduction of traffic accidents, the need for better health indicators, and for improved methods of screening sample populations for early signs of disease or for incapacity. These needs are requiring and justifying more effort than they are currently getting.

The most important channel through which developing countries can obtain new health technology is technology transfer usually mediated by industry. At the user end there must exist the necessary infrastructure and willingness to receive the technology, provide the means to distribute and create an appropriate pattern of human and organizational performance in using, maintaining and supporting the technology. Clearly, massive educational efforts are also needed for the successful transfer of modern technology.

Future perspectives on concepts of disease

The notion of disease is rooted in folk psychology, is extremely rich in connotations and absorbs new meanings in each consecutive era of social and scientific history. The

---

[1] For details of the report of the colloquium, see *Further Reading*. The full text of the report of the colloquium can be accessed online at http://whqlibdoc.who.int/hq/1995/WHO_RPS_ACHR-CIOMS_95.pdf.

current concept of disease is polythetic, i.e. it is a class defined by any number of the following characteristics: clinical abnormalities, pathological abnormalities of structure and/or function, etiological agents, biological disadvantage and "therapeutic concern". Although disease is difficult to define, recent conceptual advances articulate the general idea of disease into more meaningful empirical components. The triad "disease-illness-sickness" is useful in social research while the triad "impairment-disability-handicap" is the basis for the WHO classification (ICIDH). In general the current tendency is one towards a multidimensional or multiaxial conceptualization of disease phenomena which includes several relatively independent dimensions: clinical syndromes, structural functional abnormalities, etiology, co-morbidity and social functioning. There are considerable advantages in the operationalization of diagnosis and in clinical measurement in the individual case. The reliability of diagnosis is improving due to the development of standard diagnostic criteria and there is a clear trend of applying decision-making theory and epidemiological databases to the clinical diagnostic process.

At the population level, diagnosis and measurement are applied in the context of epidemiology which maps diseases in terms of incidence and prevalence, lifetime risk, relative and attributable risks, mortality and standard mortality rates, DALY (disability adjusted life years) and QALY (quality of life adjusted years).

Some of the problems that have to be solved by society are: dimensional versus categorical definitions of diseases. With the increasing capacity to diagnose preclinical disease and predictive testing, we are faced with serious ethical, social and economic dilemmas. There is a tendency for the conceptual boundaries between disease and non-disease to become blurred and to massively increase the medicalization of social problems. There is a need for a common language and worldwide agreement on operational definition of impairments, disabilities, and handicaps and the use of multidimensional constructs in distinguishing disease from health. Furthermore, there is a need for a new partnership of science and ethics based on the concept of "beneficiaries in trust".

Public health and the economic environment

Nineteen countries among forty-three LDCs show declining caloric supply per capita, while twenty-four indicate increasing caloric supply. In either case daily requirements are not met, and about 1.1 billion people in the developing world do not have sufficient income to obtain adequate energy from their diet. In particular the situation in south Asia is still serious and sub-Saharan Africa shows a definite worsening. Public expenditure on health has declined in a number of countries. Furthermore, most current public spending goes for expensive curative services benefiting mainly the rich, in contrast to inexpensive health measures, such as immunization and prenatal care. Among the key success elements of countries that have grown fast and achieved low levels of poverty and better health, the following were identified: investment in education, outward orientation, reliance on markets, selective governmental interventions, asset redistribution, and technology transfer. Improved criteria for allocating and channelling foreign assistance, and deeper understanding of the implications of automation on employment are needed. The dependency burden and its impact on who pays for health improvements needs to be clarified. Better ways to reduce unfavourable health effects during the epidemiological transition must be sought. The investigation of nutritional and household factors as well as levels of information available in countries in close geographical relationship might be important. The DALY methodology should be critically evaluated.

Public health and the constructed environment

Humankind's ability to maintain and even improve its health depends on being able to cope with the physical and chemical risks imposed by an increasingly difficult and hostile environment, which consists of chemical, microbial, physical, biological, economic, social and psycho-mental components forming a complex ecosystem. These risks include pollution of the air, surface and ground water, the food chain and contamination of the general environment by ionizing radiation and electromagnetic fields. Public health has to be concerned with the development of environmental medicine with increases in chronic low level exposures.

A research agenda for the future was proposed which would provide the information necessary to develop programmes and public health measures to meet these emerging issues. The agenda should include:

— human health assessment (correlation of environmental changes with the health of human beings under a variety of conditions and belonging to different age and ethnic groups);
— global environmental epidemiology (investigation of environmentally-induced changes in health linked to changes in natural eco-systems and ambient environmental exposure);
— ecosystem dynamics in relation to health;
— integrated chemical and biological monitoring and environmental engineering;
— systems research (planning and organization of environmental research at global level).

The importance of the interaction between the natural and the social environment is considered of crucial importance thus requiring concentrated research. Increasing industrial growth and centralization have led to population migrations, areas of massive pollution with associated social problems of consumerism and unemployment. Unemployment may well be the greatest problem facing the world in the next century and must be considered a health hazard because of the social problems it creates.

Public health and societal behaviour

Exploring the parameters of the health transition (the nature of the epidemiological change, the role of family members in recognition and action, and responsiveness of health transitional problems) needs to be extended across the full range of transitional problems. This approach should be included among the priorities for future research, including the special concerns that ways and means be developed for facilitating the incorporation of research findings into relevant health systems development. Health services research focused on population-based, equity-oriented, primary health care located in different socioeconomic, cultural and political settings must be expanded. It is of special concern that the incorporation of research findings into relevant health systems be realized in various developmental settings. It is increasingly appreciated that communities have critical roles to play in national development. One of the goals of primary health care is to involve communities in ways that empower them for their own further development. Carefully built partnerships are necessary between communities and health care providers if the goal of empowerment with impact is to be reached. There are no universal solutions or blueprints for primary health care and community involvement. Adaptation to local needs, ingenuity and resources are required.

A partnership in health policy formulation is necessary. In the past policy-makers and researchers worked in separate worlds which led to suboptimal or even undesirable results. In a partnership between researchers and governmental health policy-makers both work together in formulating the questions, considering research approaches and examining the results and in formulating and implementing the policies. Wider studies of how policies are made and implemented should be encouraged.

Advances in science bring challenges to the ethical understanding of health problems and interventions to improve health and this understanding varies according to the value system of a society. Ethics have a critical role in guiding the construction of policies. But there are tensions between what is desirable in terms of both ethics and policy and what is possible in the face of resource constraints. A growing capacity for ethical analysis as well as sensitivity to linking ethics with policy formulation is needed in all societies.

There are many important advances in public health that are well supported by research but are lacking widespread acceptance and implementation. There should be strong initiatives to identify such failures of implementation and to develop strategies for remedying the problem. These efforts to identify failures and implement important advances should involve joint efforts of scientists, policymakers, health systems leaders, educators, community representatives and other interested parties.

It is important to realize that advances in science that are particularly relevant to health and social development can rarely be directly applied to recipient countries. They need to be adapted, absorbed and modified, and local people and their organizations must be prepared for effective utilization. Capacity building for more effective partnership in transfers and uses of such advances are a central feature of national development. Thus careful attention must be given by developed countries and international organization to building the capacities of developing countries for more effective partnership in the generation and utilization of advances that are relevant to the health of the public.

Epilogue

Since World War II, overall population health levels have dramatically improved, as indicated by increasing life expectancies and decreasing infant mortality rates. Much of this progress has been due to improvements in economic conditions, education and nutrition, to widespread programmes in vaccination and immunization, and to more effective therapeutic procedures particularly in the area of infectious diseases. However, excessive population growth remains a major problem and the gap between wealthy and poor nations is widening. In many of the poorer developing nations nutritional levels are decreasing.

The dichotomy between health and disease is deeply rooted in human history but cannot be unequivocally defined. The WHO definition of health as a state of complete physical, psychological and social well-being (and not merely of the absence of disease and infirmity) is conceptually sound but indicators for "Quality of Life" must still be developed. Earlier attempts by Breslow and his group and by Bush and his group have never been fully accepted. Based on extensive interviews, Breslow established indicators for the physical, mental and societal health for the population of Alameda County in California in 1965 and 1974. Measuring health at two points in time he could assess changes in health in this population but he refrained from any predictions. Bush established an elaborate scale of disability, ranging from death to complete health but never tested his concept on a large scale. In 1993 the World Bank published its annual world development report with the focus on health problems. They proposed disability adjusted life years (DALY) as a measure of the burden of disease and applied this concept to express the health level for different age and sex groups of the eight regions of the world. This represents a gargantuan effort which at this time is doomed to failure since the necessary data are simply not available. Nevertheless it is a welcome initiative by a powerful organization which may lead to better and more reliable databases. It is not always realized how unreliable official data are. For example, despite its elaborate census system the under count of the population in the USA had increased from an estimated 1% in 1980 to 4% (or 10 million) in 1990. In particular the development of population or region specific epidemiological databases will be needed in support of new diagnostic technologies.

There is a rapid increase in conditions which were not considered diseases in earlier times but for which interventions are now available. This has led to a blurring of the conceptual boundaries between disease and "non-disease" which is responsible for the rise in medicalizing social problems. This difficulty must be faced, particularly if one considers the limits of available societal and economic resources, as has been so well expressed by Garrett Harding in "The Tragedy of the Commons".

On the other hand moral and ethical considerations demand equal access to health care for all, independent of economic, racial or sexual differences. In order to achieve such a goal, health care systems must be restructured in such a way that permits cheap and high quality health care at some minimum level for all. The World Bank estimates that such a package consisting of public health measures and essential clinical services would cost between 12 dollars per capita for low income countries to 22 dollars per capita for middle income countries and would reduce the total disease burden by about 25%. Although these estimated costs represent only a small percentage of the average per capita income, very large fractions of these populations live far below the poverty level and would be unable to raise even minimal amounts of funds for health care since they are unable even to purchase sufficient food.

Participants to the colloquium recognized the real and urgent need to mobilize the scientific communities to devote more attention than hither to the development, application and implementation of scientific advances for health and human development. They suggested the creation of a forum for the scientific community to discuss the needs and implementation of research necessary for global health development by WHO and CIOMS. CIOMS has a special mission to fulfil in continuing to perform its advocacy role for international order and a code of ethics in health research.

Annex 8
Summary of the 1998 Research policy agenda for science and technology to support global health development (excerpts)[1]

A view to possible futures

As it enters the third millennium, the world finds itself facing great challenges, in spite of the fact that there have been unexpected but remarkable worldwide changes in politics and economics. Whereas the use of advanced technologies is providing people with new opportunities, there is an increase in starvation and misery in many countries. In addition, prosperity, human culture and human rights are being seriously threatened by a lack of control over population growth, destruction of the environment, the over-consumption of non-renewable resources and an accelerating process of demand-stimulating innovation. One option, of course, could be "laissez faire", that is, to let things take their course, solving problems piecemeal, and hopefully not too late. The "Research Policy Agenda" takes a different view.

It is becoming clear that present attitudes and paths to development must change. Certain development trends have to be redirected, or even reversed, and then embedded in new sustainable processes. Humankind must identify solutions which allow the transformation of dangerous trends and which will involve the accommodation of conflicting goals. A new kind of "global rationality" has to be developed and accepted. A fair distribution of resources, wealth and social security should be the cornerstones for future politics. The world needs a "contract" between societies to accept globally the principles of equity and solidarity and to implement a sustainable way of living for the future. In such a contract WHO and the scientific community should assume a prominent role and should accept their specific responsibilities. The ACHR system has recognized these challenges and initiated the preparation of this document on the contribution of science and technology with specific emphasis on global health development. "A Research policy agenda for science and technology to support global health development" is intended to lead on to an ongoing research planning process and an implementation methodology.

The vision of the Research Policy Agenda is one of global cooperation between the scientific community, governments, non-governmental organizations and all partners in public health, in an innovative approach that will "make a difference" – a profound difference – in the health status of the world in the 21st Century.

In essence the Agenda advocates the timely sensitivity to evolving problems of critical significance to global health, the mobilization of and support to scientific networks

---

[1] For details of the *Research policy agenda*, see ref. 19. The full text can be accessed online at http://whqlibdoc.who.int/hq/1998/WHO_RPS_ACHR_98.1.pdf.

for solving problems through systematic research, and the effective communication of research findings to decision-makers. The premises underlying the Agenda include the recognition that:

1. In spite of diversity, there is a common fate, condition and ethic of all humanity that unifies action for global health development.
2. While most health impacts are "local", many underlying causes and potential solutions are "global" and multifactorial in nature.
3. Global health challenges, problems and determinants call for a more systematic global approach in support of action at international, national and local levels.
4. The world's scientists and scientific institutions must work together and with all relevant partners, not only in conventional "biomedical research", but in all research that contributes to health.
5. "Intelligent" research networks need to be expanded or developed around major issues, taking advantage of appropriate communications technologies.
6. A continuous process for definition, planning, implementation and evaluation of global research imperatives and opportunities is required.

"Globalization" or a world "system"?

It is increasingly and commonly argued that new global forces have eroded national borders facilitating the transfer of goods, services, people, values and lifestyles from one country to another. Socio-cultural, political and even religious influences, as well as economic, ecological and behavioural factors are perceived as shaping the future world order. "Globalization of trade, technology and travel" are quoted as important new phenomena with direct relevance to world health. Yet, interdependence between sectors and countries has been under investigation for several decades, including, for example, the "Club of Rome" studies. Is it possible to model the system?

Computer simulation models have been developed in an attempt to predict the behaviour of the entire world system. They have been characterized by a high degree of aggregation, based on a few variables: capital investment, population, food production, non-renewable resources and pollution. Early models predicted that an equilibrium state sustainable into the future was only possible if industrial output as well as population were limited through growth regulation policies and if technological policies were instituted assuring resource recycle, pollution control, increased lifetime of all forms of capital and restoration of eroded and infertile soil. In those models, the health sector was largely disregarded.

It must be recalled that a social system is characterized by organized complexity and extensive subsystem interdependencies within the system's boundaries, Systems analysis permits to identify inputs, outputs and systems parameters and classify them within a hierarchical framework. Goals can be defined and a hierarchy of values established. In principle, resources can be assessed and allocated and priorities established within the framework of the overall system. Based on that, a rational search for solutions can be initiated and objectives and programme activities can be properly articulated.

One of the major problems is the quantification of a system's variables. Conventionally, many social indicators are expressed in monetary terms, thus associating happiness with material welfare. National data collection and analysis based on averages are not geared towards identifying local pockets of poverty or poor health conditions, despite the impact such pockets may have on overall performance. The use of the GNP of the poorest 40% of the population (GNP40) as a measure of income distribution has been proposed and the ratio of GNP40/GNP for typical developing countries has been found to be in the range of 0.17 to 0.41. Perhaps other measurements are needed to more fully capture the complexity of disparities, sub-system relationships and concepts of human welfare.

A pioneering effort performed in the late seventies investigated the relationships between seven socioeconomic subsystems in a cross-national and cross-temporal study of 29 developed and 25 developing countries. The sectors considered as subsystems included demography, health, medical resources, nutrition, education, housing, communication and economy. The performance of these subsectors showed that certain changes could be closely correlated until a particular level of development was reached, then would vary at different rates. The ranking of all the countries along a socioeconomic and a health dimension showed that economy (a social dimension consisting of housing, nutrition and medical resources), health and education contribute most to the rank order of developing countries, while a social dimension consisting of communication, housing and education assumed that role for developed countries. Although many countries in both groups showed relatively balanced development with respect to the socioeconomic and the health dimensions, two special groups could be identified as either "health efficient" or "health inefficient". Such analyses clearly represent the type of conceptualization which could contribute to a better understanding of global systems dynamics in world health.

The mission of WHO in research

Mandate

WHO has a clear constitutional mandate to "promote and conduct research in the field of health" (Constitution of the World Health Organization, Article 2n). WHO has recently reaffirmed that it "will continue to promote and support health research and technological development in accordance with its policies and in response to the health problems in countries. It will identify important bioethical issues in certain aspects of health research and in their clinical applications, and will stimulate the exchange of opinion and the sharing of information in that regard. It will stimulate and support the strengthening of health research capacity in countries, with emphasis on affordability and sustainability. By monitoring and analysing advances in medical, biological and behavioural sciences and health technology it will seek to identify existing technology that could be used directly or be further developed to solve significant problems in health care; to assess new and emerging science and technology for future application in solving health problems; and to catalyze research to meet known and emerging needs." Also: "It will strengthen the collection, assessment and dissemination of information on cost-effective new methods for health development. It will explore mew ways of intensifying cooperation with the scientific community and promoting more active involvement and collaboration." (WHO Ninth General Programme of Work, para. 64, 65).

Health research strategy

Prior to adopting the 9th WHO Global Programme of Work, the World Health Assembly, in 1990, called for a clearly enunciated health research strategy in order to translate the research goals, priorities and programmes into coherent and coordinated action in support of health for all (resolution WHA43.19). To fulfil this, the ACHR, drawing on the work of its own task forces and subcommittees, considered that new dimensions were needed to give proper emphasis to the infrastructural, economic, environmental and socio-behavioural aspects of the health research strategy given in 1986. That previous health research strategy, known as the McKeown report, had interpreted the goal of "health for all by the year 2000" as aiming to achieve a substantial improvement in health in all countries, particularly those where the need is greatest. It stressed that " it is not unrealistic to define more precisely a level of health below which it is hoped that no country will fall: infant mortality below 50 (per 1000 live births) and life expectation at birth of 60 years." These levels were reached in the middle of this century by the developed countries and more recently in some developing countries.

The determinants of the global health picture were also described and the consequential approaches to research planning were discussed, based on the following key observations:

- The human genetic constitution was much the same today as it was a hundred thousand years ago, before the advent of any form of pastoral or agricultural activity. That is to say, we now face vastly changed conditions of life with the same genetic equipment of our ancestors who were hunter-gatherers.
- The modern transformation of health in developed countries and the associated increase of populations, which began more than a century before effective medical intervention was possible, was to be attributed largely to improvements in living conditions.
- Research had shown us the nature of infectious disease and the possibility of its prevention by environmental measures and immunization.
- It had been recognized in the last few decades that most non-communicable diseases could be prevented by changes in living conditions and behaviour; the most striking evidence was the recent decline of coronary deaths.

In 1986 it was considered that countries with very limited resources should give higher priority to research and services in nutrition, immunization and sanitation.

In order to further elaborate the formulation of a WHO health research strategy, ACHR drew on the work of its own subgroups, namely, the Task Forces on Science and Technology, on Health Development Research, on Evolving Problems of critical Significance to Health, and the Sub-committees on Health and the Economy and on Research Capability Strengthening. The ACHR considered that although the Health Research Strategy adopted in 1988 remained a valid cornerstone of WHO's research strategy, new dimensions should be added to give proper emphasis to infrastructural, economic, environmental and behavioural aspects. The revised strategy focused on: the relevance of health and the economy, global problems and global solutions, health research and human development, science and technology policies, the emergence of new ethical issues and research capability strengthening in developing countries. It further emphasized: a world in transition, the changing scene of science and technology and the importance of identifying research needs on the basis of health needs.

"Health for All in the 21st Century"

A 1998 document entitled "Health for All in the 21st Century" discussed the role of WHO in fostering the use of, and innovation in, science and technology. It stated that advances in science and technology have yielded substantial dividends to health in the past.

Scientific and technological progress is likely to yield even greater benefits for all in the twenty-first century. Rapid progress in several fields over the next decades should allow poorer countries to take maximal advantage of developments in technology and benefit from the experiences of other countries. Information and Communication Technology (ICT), for instance, offers opportunities for the most remote researchers to access critical information and to participate fully in scientific progress.

Global research efforts should be directed towards areas where substantial gains are needed for health. These are complemented by country-specific research priorities and action, through which countries will work towards improved national and global health. It was concluded that global areas of concentration should include research that:

— identifies social, environment and specific sectoral policies and actions that advance health;
— informs health policy and improves health equity;
— evaluates the effectiveness of interventions to reduce inequities in health;
— maximizes health systems efficiency and leads to sustainable health systems;
— accelerates the reduction of childhood disease, malnutrition, and maternal and perinatal mortality;
— addresses changing microbial threats and develops strategies for their prevention and control;
— identifies effective preventive, promotive and curative approaches to non-communicable diseases and health consequences of aging; and
— leads to control of violence and injuries.

Closer partnerships between science and technology, between users and innovators, and between the private and public sectors will increase the chances that innovations in science will contribute to improved health worldwide through the development of technology and the implementation of research. The scope of technologies for health extends from those that provide a direct benefit to health such as genetic modification, biologicals, pharmaceuticals and medical devices, to those that are supportive of health systems functions, such as telecommunications, information technologies, devices for environmental protection and food technologies.

It was concluded that in assessing and promoting new technologies for health, the following should be considered: their ability to contribute to life and health; to promote equity; to respect privacy and individual autonomy and the extent to which they focus on the determinants of health. At the same time, an effort must be made to adopt a long timeframe and a wide view, as the benefits and applications of technology are not always immediately understood, realized, or affordable.

Meeting the global challenge by science and technology

It must be recalled that the global resources for science and technology are very substantial. The market economies (about 75% of the world) are spending approximately 2% of their GNP for research and development, i.e. of the order of half a trillion USD (including the private sector, 1997). The number of scientists and engineers worldwide exceeds 4 million (UNESCO, 1996) with a ratio between North and South ranging between 25:1 (average) and 7:1 (China). These resources are obviously unevenly distributed and not matched to problems which face the world.

The challenge is to involve all of the world's human resources, North, South, East and West, to investigate and solve global health problems by working together and exploiting modern communication technology. It is argued that research imperatives and opportunities need to be continuously identified and further developed and refined.

Global health problems call for a global approach

The first component of the Agenda is an appreciation of the need for doing comprehensive research on complex problems (not discipline-specific problems). The global health situation reveals the fact that the world is not confronted merely by health problems as such, but rather by an intricate system of interacting factors and trends, many of which do not seem (a priori) to be directly related to health. When such trends as are seen in population dynamics (growth, migration, urbanization industrialization, environmental degradation, (human) behaviour, and changing value systems) are studied, not in isolation but in interwoven human systems, then it becomes feasible to devise solutions within the boundaries of realistic constraints. Best seen as constantly evolving problems of critical significance to global health, these are at the core of health development.

The world's scientists must work together

The second component is based on the recognition that while the world boasts a large and increasingly skilled cadre of scientists and technological experts, the skills and experiences of these individuals have, up to this point, not been sufficiently recruited to solve global health problems. Scientists, particularly those in the world's many universities, rarely conduct joint research into what are often less than "cutting edge" topics, e.g. better procedures for food safely, water quality, infant care, immunization, etc. This aspect of the Agenda consists in harnessing the power of science, technology and medicine, and calls on the world's scientific community to combine their, hitherto often fragmented, efforts in the direction of research for "global" problem solving.

Intelligent research networks will be required

The third part of the agenda is the networking of global scientific brain-power in small, intelligent research networks (or "IRENEs"). It is proposed to use Information and Communication Technology (ICT) for the establishment and coordination of a worldwide "network of scientific networks". The global ACHR has already developed the prototype for the central node of this "meta network": a planning network for health research.